Update in Geriatrics

Edited by Somchai Amornyotin

Published in London, United Kingdom

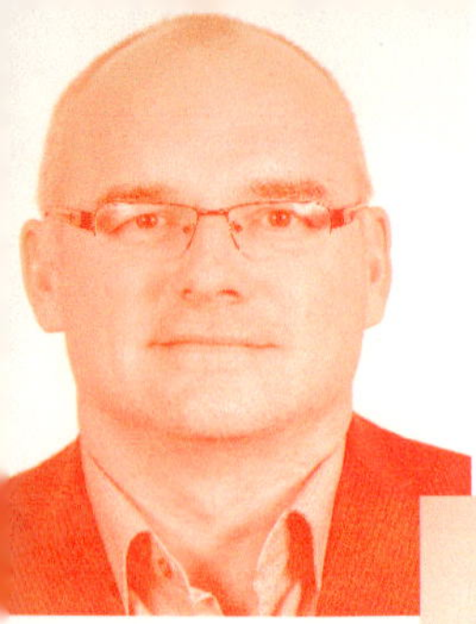
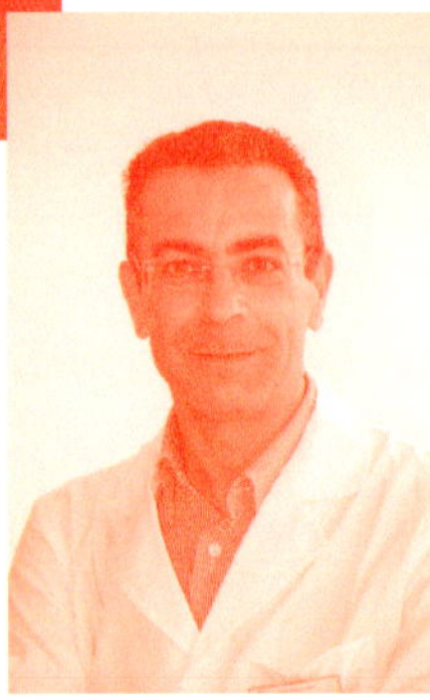
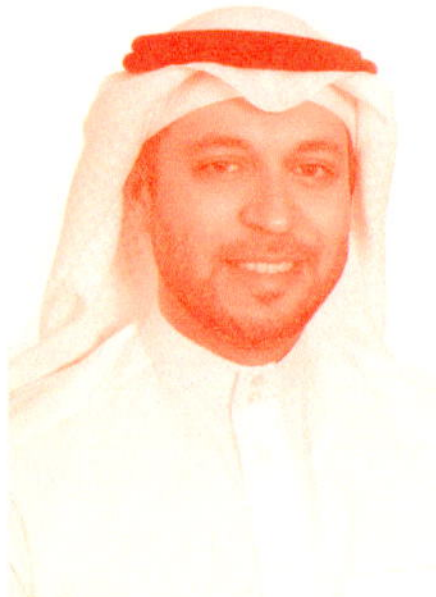
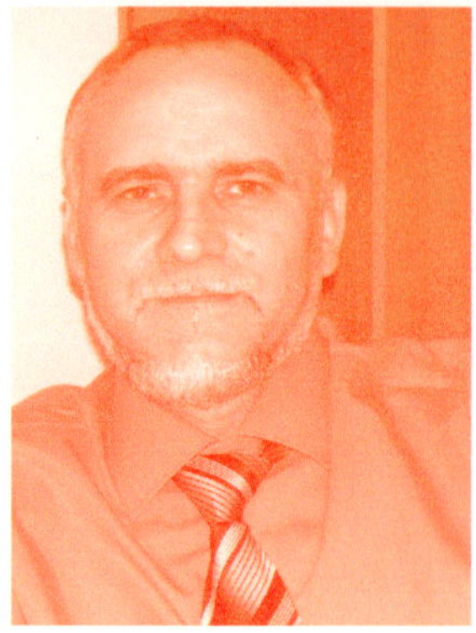
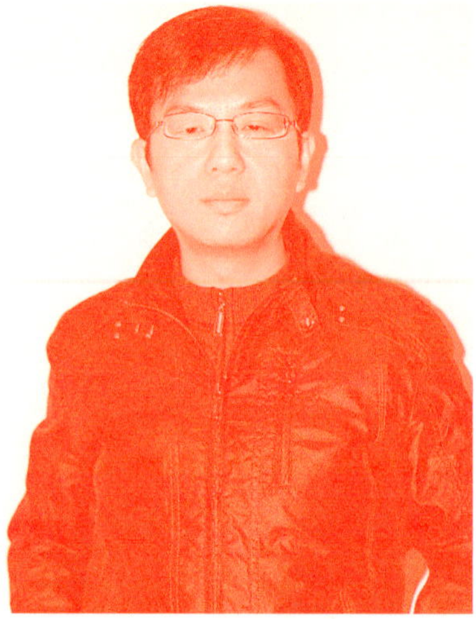
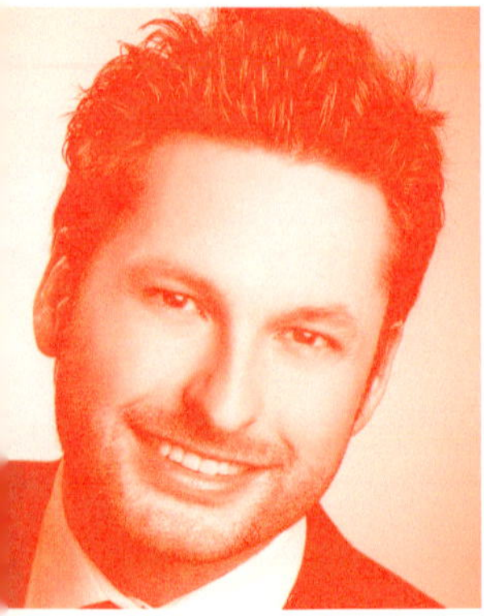
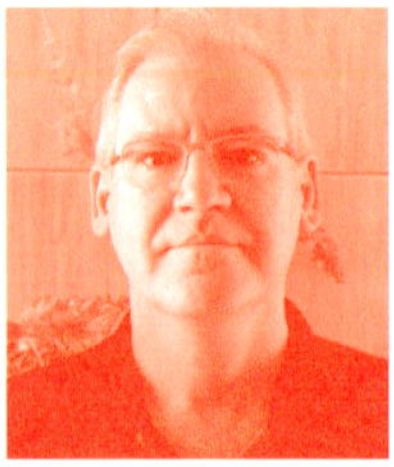

IntechOpen

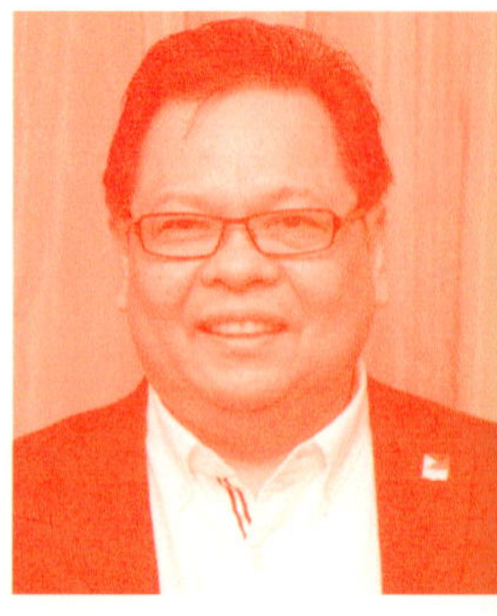
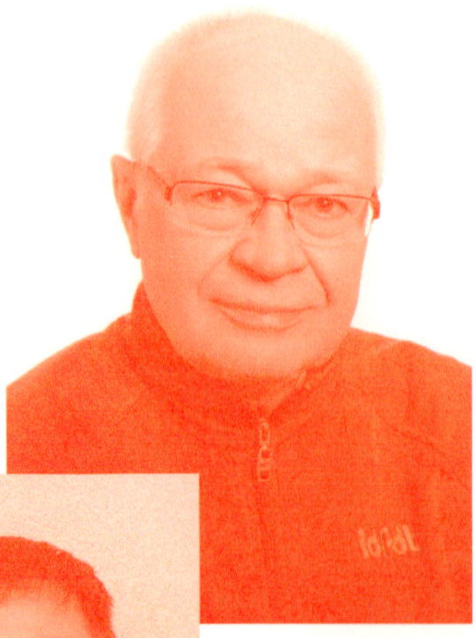
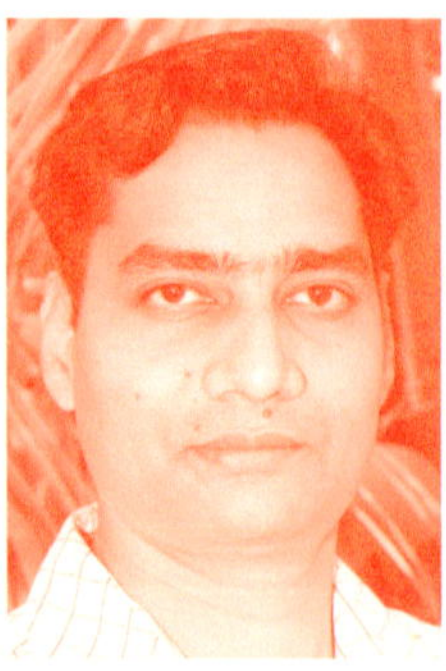
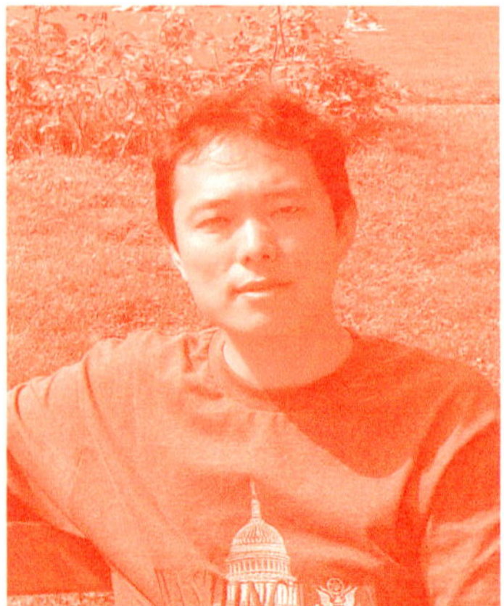
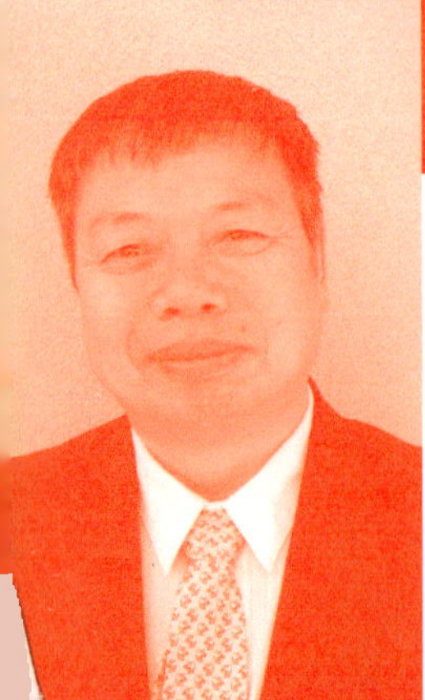
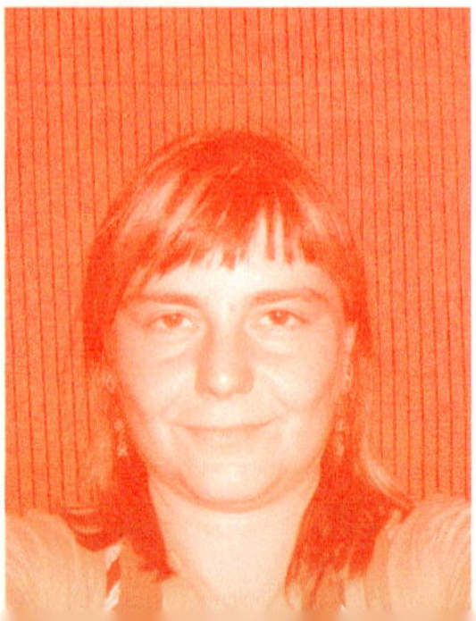

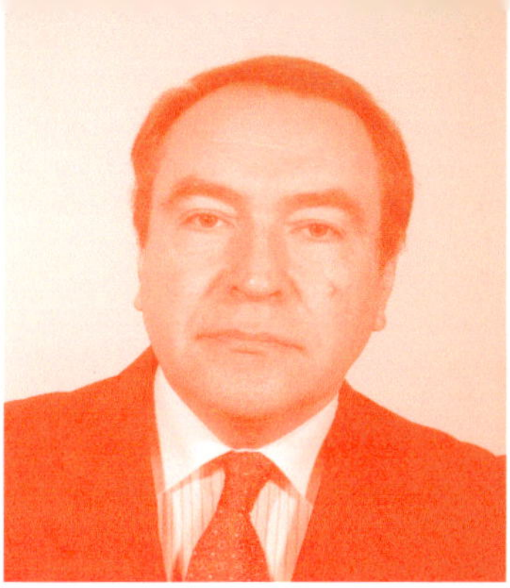
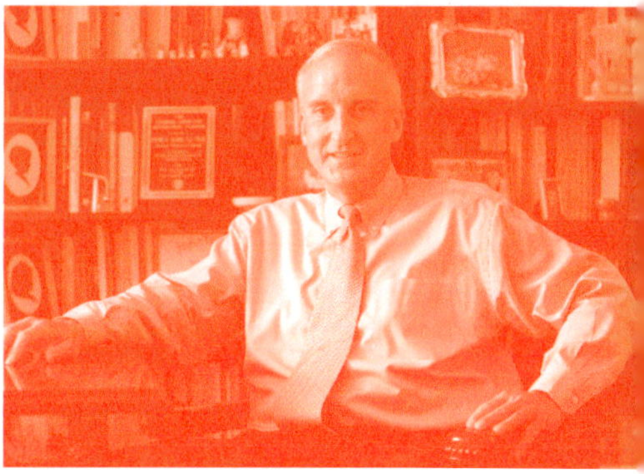
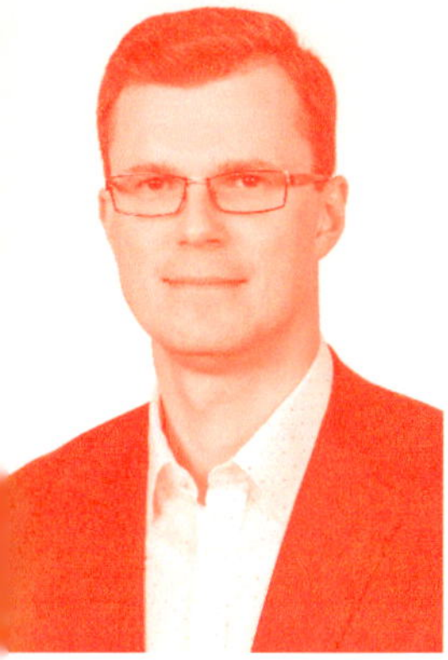
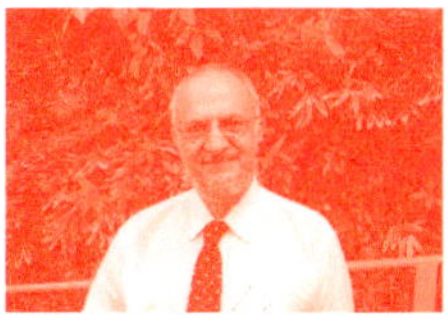
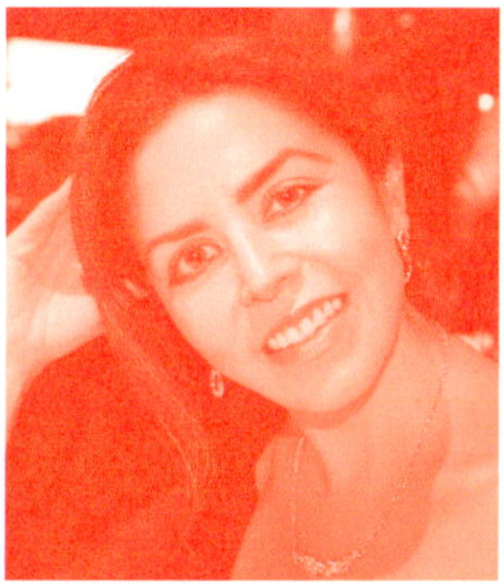

Supporting open minds since 2005

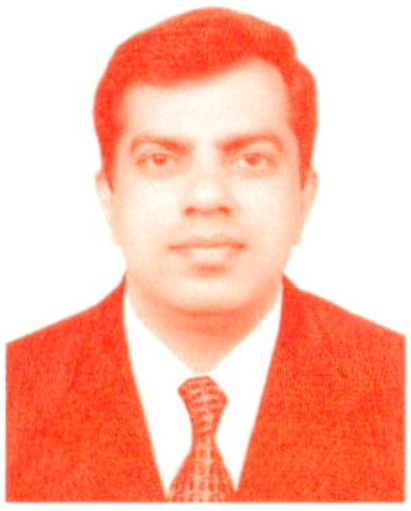
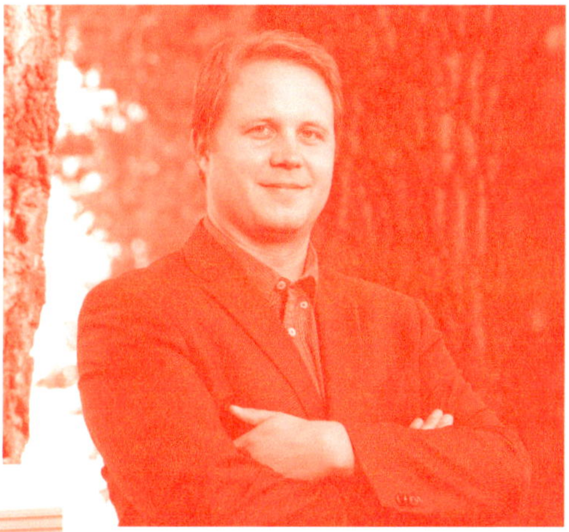
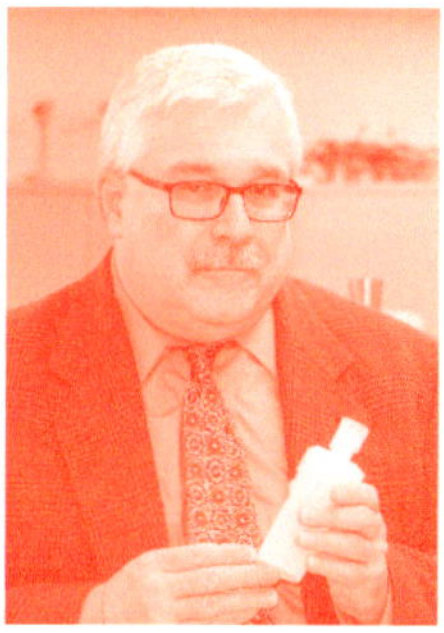
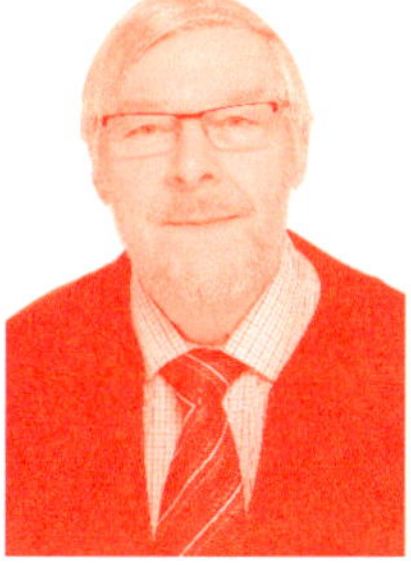
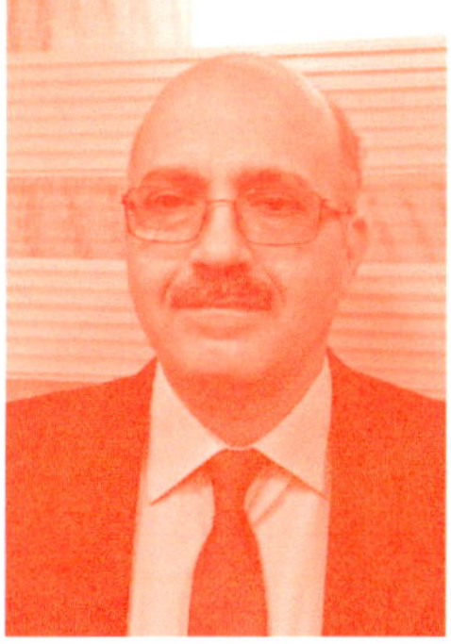
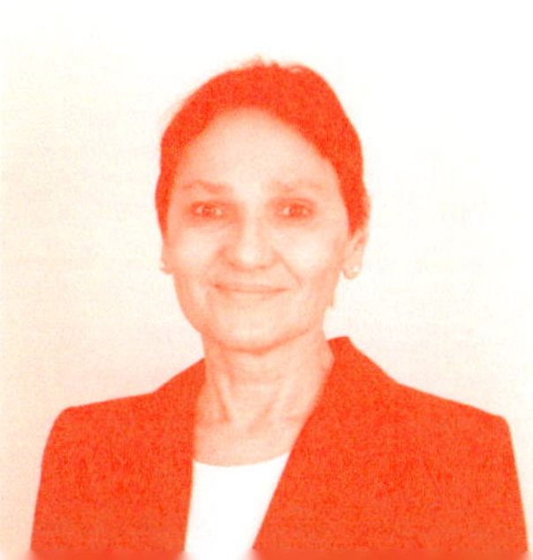
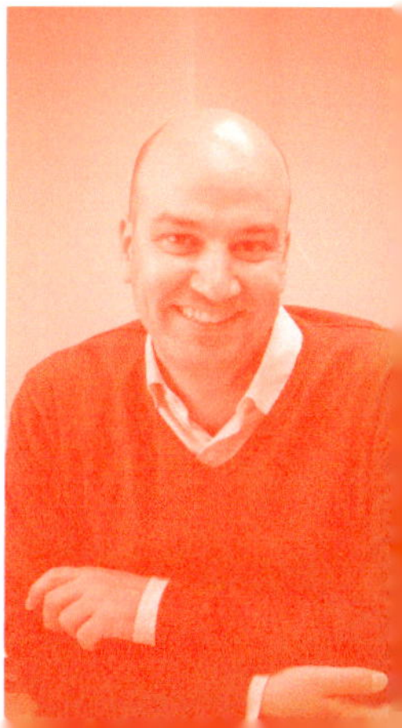

Update in Geriatrics
http://dx.doi.org/10.5772/intechopen.87300
Edited by Somchai Amornyotin

Contributors
Monica Trif, Alexandru Vasile Rusu, Berta María Álvarez Penedo, Ann-Kristin Schwarze, Wilfred Luis Clamor, Abel Toledano-González, Donna M. Lisi, Melissa O'Connor, Kaushik Nag, Nabarun Karmakar, Anjan Datta, Ana Fajreldines, Marcelo Pellizzari, Stefanía Barberis, Belen Beldarrain, Marisa Bazzano, Dabota Yvonne Yvonne Buowari, Alexander V. Panov, Marina Darenskaya, Sergey Ivanovich Kolesnikov, Sergey Dikalov, Hassan M. Heshmati, Somchai Amornyotin, Manjit Kaur Rana, Amrit Pal Singh Rana

First published in London, United Kingdom, 2021 by IntechOpen
IntechOpen is the global imprint of INTECHOPEN LIMITED, registered in England and Wales, registration number: 11086078, 5 Princes Gate Court, London, SW7 2QJ, United Kingdom
Printed in Croatia

British Library Cataloguing-in-Publication Data
A catalogue record for this book is available from the British Library

Additional hard and PDF copies can be obtained from orders@intechopen.com

Update in Geriatrics
Edited by Somchai Amornyotin
p. cm.
Print ISBN 978-1-83962-308-0
Online ISBN 978-1-83962-309-7
eBook (PDF) ISBN 978-1-83962-313-4

For EU product safety concerns:
IN TECH d.o.o., Prolaz Marije Krucifikse Kozulić 3, 51000 Rijeka, Croatia, info@intechopen.com or visit our website at intechopen.com.

Meet the editor

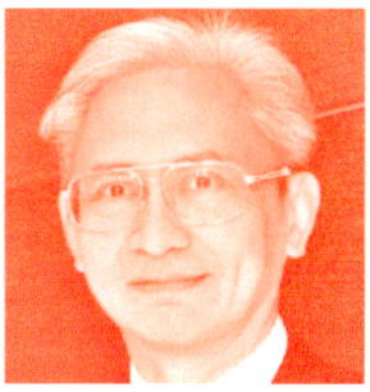

Dr. Somchai Amornyotin graduated from the Faculty of Medicine Siriraj Hospital, Mahidol University, Bangkok, Thailand, in 1989. He joined the staff of the Department of Anesthesiology, Faculty of Medicine Siriraj Hospital, Mahidol University, in 1996. In 2020, he became a professor in the Department of Anesthesiology, Faculty of Medicine Siriraj Hospital, Mahidol University. His first scientific paper was published in Thailand in 1999. He has practiced anesthesia since 2002. More than eighty of his research articles have been published in Thai and international medical journals. Dr. Amornyotin is a member of the Royal College of Anesthesiologists of Thailand, the Gastroenterological Association of Thailand, and many scientific societies. He is also a reviewer and editor for many international journals.

Contents

Preface

Geriatrics is a topic of great interest in medicine and among the general public. In several countries, the increase in life expectancy has made the elderly the fastest-growing segment of the population. The numbers of geriatric persons are increasing worldwide, which means there will also be an increase in their health needs as well. The geriatric population experiences significant alterations of numerous organ systems as a result of the aging process. They also have several co-morbidities including hypertension, cardiac disease, diabetes, cerebrovascular disease, and renal dysfunction, to name a few.

The geriatric population is quickly growing and living longer, and thus surgical demand for both elective and emergent cases is estimated to increase significantly. Caring for geriatric patients is complicated, requiring a balance between physiological and psychological alterations. Geriatric patients are vulnerable and especially sensitive to the stress of trauma, surgery, and anesthesia.

Written by experts in the field, this book presents practical knowledge of geriatrics from multiple points of view. I would like to thank these experts for their contributions. I am also grateful to IntechOpen and Mr. Mateo Pulko for their help in publishing this book.

Somchai Amornyotin MD, FRCAT
Professor,
Department of Anesthesiology,
Faculty of Medicine Siriraj Hospital,
Mahidol University,
Bangkok, Thailand

Section 1

General Aspects

Chapter 1

The Centenarians: An Emerging Population

Hassan M. Heshmati

Abstract

Long life is a topic of great interest in medicine and among the general public. The "successful aging" which is a high priority for individuals and societies, is aging without any disabilities and severe diseases. In several countries, the increase in life expectancy has led the very old to become the fastest growing segment of the population. Centenarians are subjects living 100 years or older. The majority of centenarians are females (female to male ratio around 3.6/1). A very small fraction of centenarians (up to 0.5%) will live 110 years or older (supercentenarians). Most centenarians have managed to avoid, postpone, or overcome the important age-related and life-threatening diseases and disabilities (e.g., ischemic heart disease, stroke, chronic obstructive pulmonary disease, cancer, respiratory infection, type 2 diabetes, osteoporosis, and dementia). Some forecasts suggest that most babies born in developed countries since 2000 will become centenarians. In 2020, the number of centenarians in the world was approximately 573,000, mainly from the United States of America (USA). This number could reach approximately 3,676,000 by 2050. In the absence of the genetic predisposition to become centenarian, there are several ways to extend longevity (e.g., lifestyle, reduction of several life-threatening diseases and disabilities, hormonal replacement or blockade, antioxidants, maintenance of a proper autophagic activity, stem cell therapy, and gene therapy). The continuous increase of the number of centenarians has worldwide practical implications including profound impact on intergenerational interactions and significant financial challenges for any society, especially in relation to medical expenses.

Keywords: centenarians, supercentenarians, longevity, genetics, emerging population

1. Introduction

Long life is a topic of great interest in medicine and among the general public. In several countries, the increase in life expectancy has led the very old to become the fastest growing segment of the population [1–4]. Centenarians are subjects living 100 years or older. Most centenarians have managed to avoid, postpone, or overcome the important age-related and life-threatening diseases [3, 5, 6].

The continuous increase of the number of centenarians has worldwide practical implications including profound impact on intergenerational interactions and significant financial challenges for any society, especially in relation to medical expenses.

2. Aging and lifespan

Aging is a natural universal phenomenon affecting all living organisms (e.g., plants, animals, and humans). It is a progressive deterioration of the cell and organ functioning due to damage accumulation over time. The exact underlying mechanisms of aging at the cellular level are not fully understood. The most popular theory is the free radical theory [7].

Lifespan is a biological characteristic of every species. However, it can be modified by mutations or by a variety of interventions (e.g., lifestyle, pharmacological, stem cell, and genetic interventions) [8–24].

Lifespan of living organisms ranges from few hours (animals) to few thousand years (plants). Phenotypic plasticity can affect the long lifespan of both plants and animals [25].

2.1 Plants

The lifespan in plants ranges from few weeks to few thousand years. Bristlecone pine (*Pinus longaeva*), a tree found in the higher mountains of California (USA), is among the plants with the longest lifespan (around 5,000 years) (**Figure 1**).

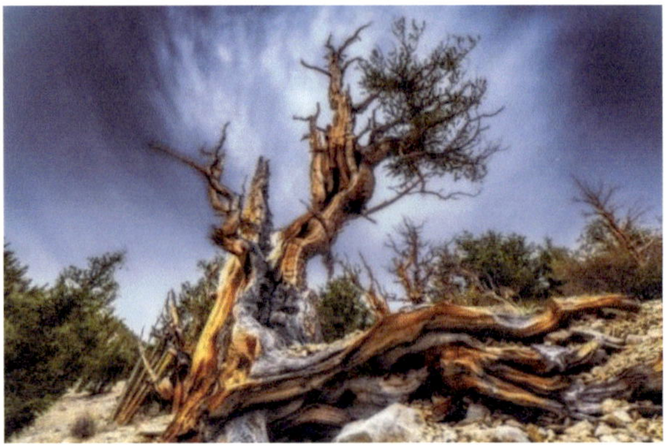

Figure 1.
Bristlecone pine (Pinus longaeva) can live around 5,000 years (Picture downloaded from the internet "Google Images").

2.2 Animals

The lifespan in animals is between few hours to few hundred years. The shortest lifespan is seen with mayfly (up to 24 hours). The longest lifespan is observed with clam (more than 400 years). Ming the clam was the oldest clams ever discovered (507 years old). Ming was accidentally killed in 2006 during a fact-finding mission (**Figure 2**).

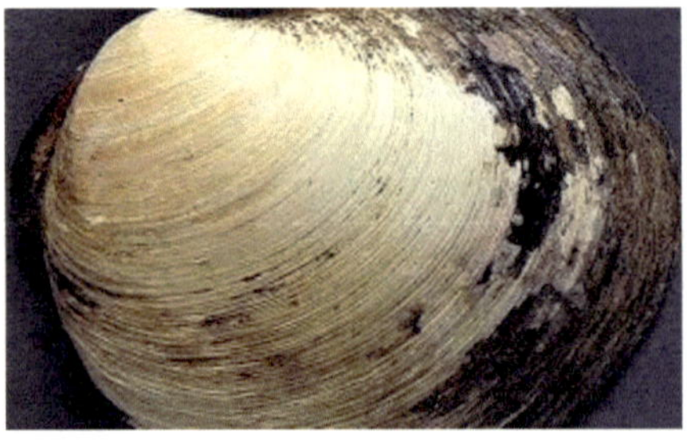

Figure 2.
Ming the clam lived 507 years (Picture downloaded from the internet "Google Images").

2.3 Humans

The theoretical lifespan in humans is around 120 years. However, very few individuals reach this theoretical age since several events can impact longevity (e.g., diseases, suicide, accident, and war).

Human aging results from accumulation of genetic, molecular, and cellular damages. It is a multifactorial process. There are several theories explaining the aging phenomenon. The most wildly accepted theory of aging is the free radical theory [7]. According to this theory, continuous, unrepaired oxidative damage of macromolecules constitutes the molecular basis of aging.

Aging and lifespan are influenced by multiple factors including genetic, epigenetic, lifestyle, environmental, metabolic, and endocrine factors [3, 8–14, 21, 26–41].

Extending longevity while keeping health and vitality has been a dream for mankind since ancient times. The "successful aging" which is a high priority for individuals and societies, is aging without any disabilities and severe diseases [42, 43]. The fountain of youth is a mythical spring capable of restoring the youth of anyone who drinks or bathes in its water (**Figure 3**).

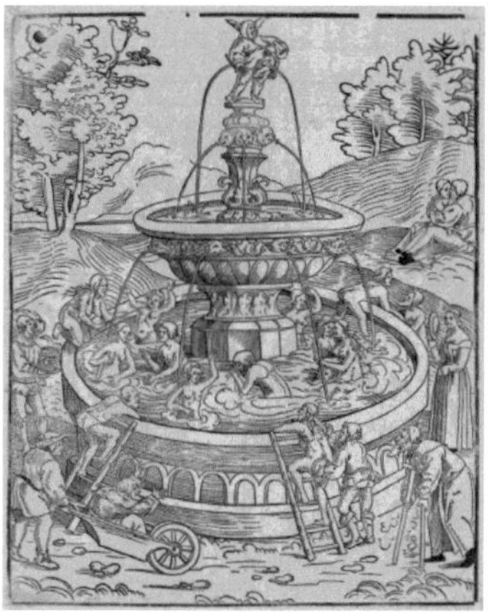

Figure 3.
The fountain of youth (from Erhard Schön, 1525) is a mythical remedy to aging (Picture downloaded from the internet "Google Images").

2.3.1 Physiological changes associated with aging

With aging, there is a gradual, time-dependent, and heterogeneous decline of physiological functions (**Figure 4**). The human body goes through multiple physiological changes including an overall decrease in the size of organs (e.g., brain shrinkage), endothelial pro-atherosclerotic changes, ovarian atrophy, osteopenia (predominantly in women), sarcopenia (mainly in the lower body), adipose tissue enlargement (mostly visceral fat), and skin atrophy (especially in women) (non-exhaustive list) [9, 10, 32, 41]. Some changes are very subtle (within normal ranges) with no or unknown clinical consequences. Lifestyle conditions (e.g., diet, exercise, and medications) and environmental factors (e.g., noise, temperature, and air quality) can delay or potentiate these changes.

Autophagy ("self-eating") is a major protein turnover pathway where cellular components are delivered into the lysosomes for degradation and recycling. It maintains cellular homeostasis under stress conditions. The autophagic activity decreases in aging individuals [21].

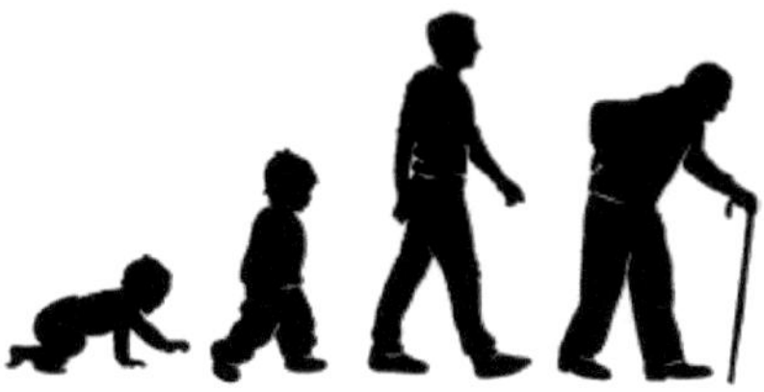

Figure 4.
Aging is associated with a gradual decline of different functions and performances (Picture downloaded from the internet "Google Images").

Mitochondria are major contributors to the maintenance of energy homeostasis. They are important sources of reactive oxygen species (ROS) generation. ROS can cause oxidation of macromolecules including DNA. Aging subjects have progressive mitochondrial decline [10, 11, 39, 44].

Aging is associated with a mild inflammatory state that is sometimes referred to as "inflammaging". This inflammatory state is characterized by increased blood levels of several adipokines (e.g., interleukin 6 and tumor necrosis factor alpha). Environmental factors can further modify the inflammatory state of aging [32].

Multiple endocrine changes occur with aging, affecting the body functions [9, 10, 12, 31, 35–37, 39–41, 45–49]. The hypothalamus, an endocrine structure located in the brain that is a master regulator of multiple hormonal secretion, plays a central role in aging. With aging, the sensitivity of the hypothalamus to different feedback signals decreases [36]. Growth hormone (GH) and insulin-like growth factor-1 (IGF-1) levels decline during aging [37]. According to most studies, free triiodothyronine (T3) levels decrease while reverse T3 (rT3) and thyroid-stimulating hormone (TSH) levels increase [45–47] with aging. Significant hormonal change occurs in women at menopause with important reduction in estrogen (E) levels [48]. In men, testosterone (T) levels decrease gradually with age [40]. There is an important decrease in dehydroepiandrosterone (DHEA) levels in aging individuals [49]. Adipose tissue, which is the largest endocrine gland, secretes several adipokines. With aging, there is an increase in the levels of most adipokines (e.g., leptin, resistin, interleukin 6, tumor necrosis factor alpha, and adiponectin) [41].

The relevant metabolic/hormonal changes during normal aging are reported in **Table 1**.

Parameter	Change
Mitochondrial activity	Decrease (gradual)
Autophagic activity	Decrease (gradual)
Inflammatory state	Increase (gradual)
GH	Decrease (gradual)
IGF-1	Decrease (gradual)
T3	Decrease (gradual)
rT3	Increase (gradual)
TSH	Increase (subtle, at old age)
E (females)	Decrease (abrupt, at menopause)
T (males)	Decrease (gradual)
DHEA	Decrease (gradual)
Adipokines	Increase (gradual)
Insulin resistance	Increase (gradual)

Table 1.
Relevant metabolic/hormonal changes during normal aging.

2.3.2 Genetic and epigenetic factors affecting aging and lifespan

Genes play an important role in the regulation of aging and lifespan [3, 8, 10, 27–29, 31, 50]. Extensive number of genes (between 300 to over 700 genes) have been listed [28, 29]. Genes include *APOE1*, *ATM*, *BCL*, *CETP*, *FOXO3A*, *HSPA*, and *TERC* (non-exhaustive list). Genetic factors that are associated with longevity are heritable [27]. Several endocrine and metabolic pathways are linked genetically with aging and contribute to different phenotypes [31]. Multiple gene mutations leading to delayed aging and increased lifespan have been discovered over the last three decades. Many of the affected genes are components of endocrine-signaling pathways (e.g., GH and IGF-1 pathways).

A dramatic example of genetic impact on aging and lifespan is observed with Hutchinson-Gilford progeria syndrome, a rare sporadic, autosomal dominant syndrome that causes premature aging. In most cases, the disorder is due to a mutation characterized by a change from glycine GGC to glycine GGT in codon 608 of exon 11 of the lamin A (*LMNA*) gene causing the production of an abnormal lamin A (progerin). Progerin accumulates in cells' nuclei and exerts multiple toxic effects [50]. The affected individuals generally die from myocardial infarction or stroke around a mean age of 15 years (**Figure 5**).

Epigenetic processes also influence aging and lifespan [8, 9, 11, 26, 30].

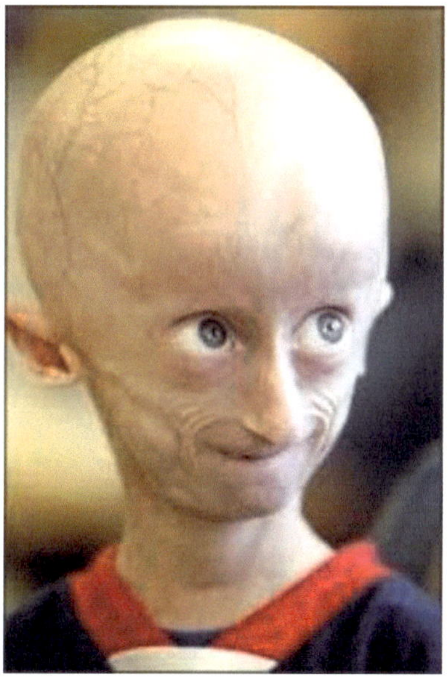

Figure 5.
Subject with premature aging due to Hutchinson-Gilford progeria syndrome (Picture downloaded from the internet "Google Images").

2.3.3 Lifestyle and environmental factors affecting aging and lifespan

Lifestyle (e.g., diet, sleep, smoking, exercise, stress, and medications) and the environment (e.g., household, social condition, noise, temperature, and air quality) play an important role in the aging process and lifespan (**Figure 6**) [8, 9, 26, 51].

Caloric restriction, physical fitness, and good air quality can delay aging and increase lifespan. Conversely, excessive food consumption, sedentary lifestyle, and air pollution will have a negative impact on aging and lifespan.

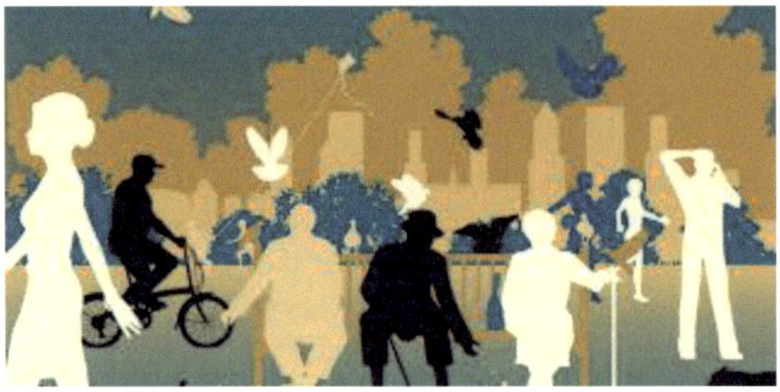

Figure 6.
Lifestyle and environmental factors can affect aging and lifespan (Picture downloaded from the internet "Google Images").

2.3.4 Metabolic factors affecting aging and lifespan

Metabolic factors play an important role in the aging process and lifespan (**Figure 7**) [10, 11, 21, 33, 34, 39, 41, 44].

The decrease in autophagic activity observed with aging contributes to accumulation of damaged macromolecules and organelles. It can aggravate age-associated diseases and, therefore, shorten lifespan [21].

Mitochondria play a key role in several theories of aging. The reduction in mitochondrial activity with aging can impact lifespan [10, 11, 39, 44].

The inflammatory state associated with aging is responsible for insulin resistance. Insulin resistance is a risk factor for the development of several chronic disorders (e.g., obesity, type 2 diabetes, and ischemic heart disease) that are influencing aging and lifespan [10, 14, 42].

The amount of body fat influences health and lifespan. Both insufficient or excess body fat as observed in subjects with underweight or overweight/obesity have been reported to be associated with increased mortality and reduced lifespan [33, 34, 41].

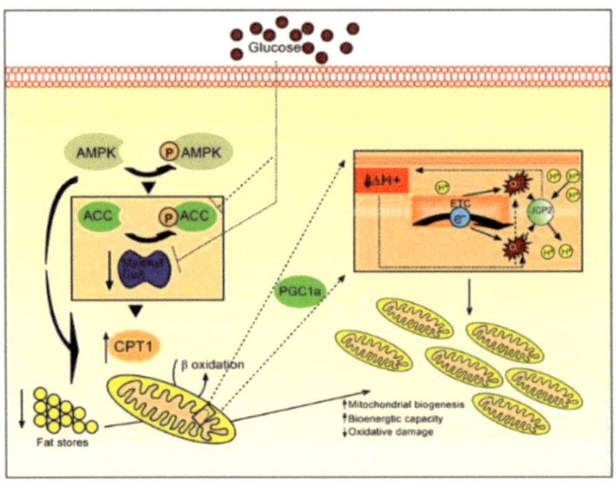

Figure 7.
Metabolic factors impact aging and lifespan (Picture downloaded from the internet "Google Images").

2.3.5 Endocrine factors affecting aging and lifespan

Hormones influence the aging process and lifespan (**Figure 8**) [9, 10, 12, 13, 31, 35–41, 45–49, 52–54]. Several endocrine-signaling changes occur during normal aging. Some hormonal changes may be beneficial while others can be harmful. The role of GH in aging and lifespan has been reported in several studies [37, 38, 52]. Reduced GH may lead to delay aging and increased lifespan while excess GH can have the opposite effects. GH secretion rate in offspring of long-lived families is lower than controls. Thyroid hormones play an important role in aging and lifespan. There is a negative correlation between thyroid hormone levels and lifespan [39]. The timing of menopause, a physiological condition occurring in women around the age of 50 years and associated with important decrease in E levels, may affect lifespan [48]. Indeed, E replacement therapy can reduce mortality (increase of lifespan) in post-menopausal women younger than 60 years [13]. In men, low T levels are associated with increased mortality [40]. Treatment with DHEA decreases insulin resistance and inflammatory adipokines and may positively impact lifespan [53]. The elevated levels of pro-inflammatory adipokines (e.g., interleukin 6 and tumor necrosis factor alpha) can negatively impact aging and lifespan. Elevated levels of adiponectin (anti-inflammatory adipokine) may be beneficial and associated with increased lifespan [41, 54].

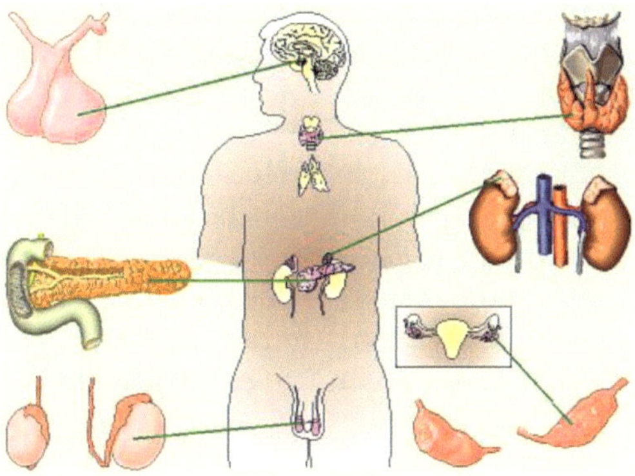

Figure 8.
Endocrine factors influence aging and lifespan (Picture downloaded from the internet "Google Images").

2.3.6 Disease occurrence with aging

The "successful aging" is aging without any disabilities and severe diseases (extension of healthspan) [42, 43]. It is more important to promote healthier aging than better treat age-related diseases.

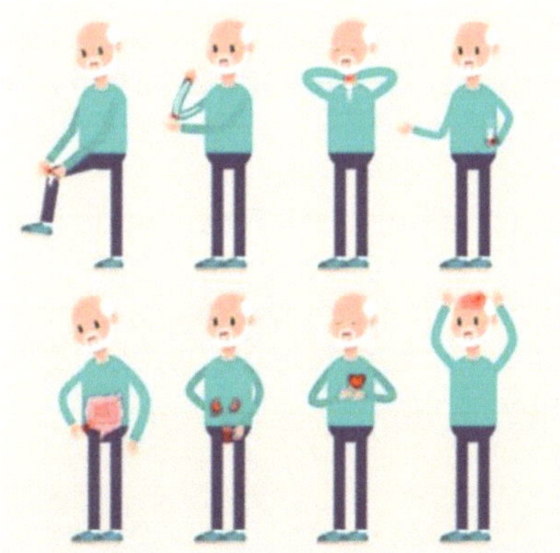

Figure 9.
Multiple organs can be affected in aging subjects (Picture downloaded from the internet "Google Images").

Several geriatric syndromes (e.g., frailty) and diseases (e.g., cardiovascular disease) occur with aging and affect quality of life and longevity [19, 42]. The incidence of adult diseases increases with age. In subjects older than 60 years, the most common age-related and life-threatening diseases and disabilities are ischemic heart disease, stroke, chronic obstructive pulmonary disease, cancer, respiratory infection, type 2 diabetes, osteoporosis, and dementia (non-exhaustive list) [14, 42]. The majority of older people may have more than one disorder. The incidence of multimorbidity (e.g., three or more diseases) increases exponentially with aging (**Figure 9**) [15]. For several of these conditions, the burden is greater in low-income and middle-income countries [42]. Some diseases (e.g., thyroid diseases) may have subtle symptoms that can be attributed to normal aging [55].

2.3.7 Life expectancy

At the beginning of the 20th century, life expectancy in most developed countries was between 45 and 50 years. Over the last several decades, there has been a gradual increase in life expectancy in most countries [27, 56]. The study of mortality and life expectancy in 195 countries and territories showed that globally, between 1950 and 2017, life expectancy increased from 48.1 years to 70.5 years for men and from 52.9 years to 75.6 years for women [56].

In less developed countries, the increase in life expectancy is mainly the result of reduced mortality at younger ages. In high-income countries, the increase in life expectancy is mainly due to rising life expectancy in subjects who are 60 years or older.

The increase in life expectancy together with the decrease in fertility rates are leading to the rapid aging of populations around the world. This has important demographic and socio-economic consequences worldwide.

3. Centenarians

Centenarians are subjects living 100 years or older. They represent a model of successful aging [3, 5, 6]. Semi-supercentenarians are those who reach an age of 105–109 years. A very small fraction of centenarians (up to 0.5%) will live 110 years or older (supercentenarians) [5, 30].

3.1 Prevalence

The total world population is currently around 7.8 billion and is projected to reach 9.9 billion by 2050. In several countries, the increase in life expectancy has led the very old to become the fastest growing segment of the population [1–4]. Some forecasts suggest that most babies born in developed countries since 2000 will become centenarians.

Estimates of the centenarian population can be difficult since some centenarians do not have birth records to confirm their age. According to United Nations estimates, in 2020, the number of centenarians in the world was approximately 573,000. This number was approximately 34,000 in 1950 and could reach approximately 3,676,000 by 2050.

3.1.1 Prevalence by gender

The majority of centenarians are females. The female to male ratio is currently around 3.6/1 and is expected to be approximately 2.9/1 by 2050 (**Figure 10**).

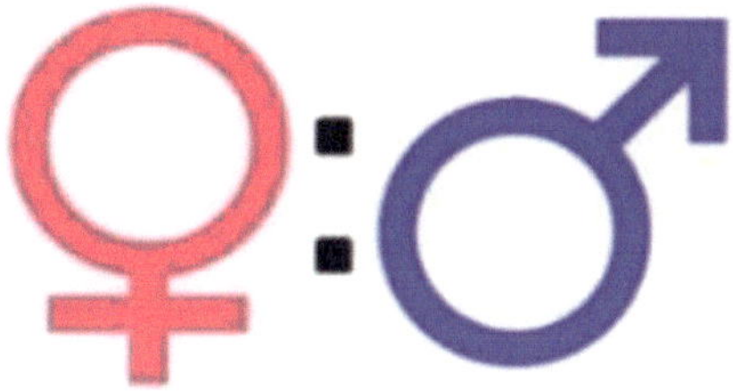

Figure 10.
Centenarians are mainly females but the female to male ratio is gradually decreasing (Picture downloaded from the internet "Google Images").

3.1.2 Prevalence by country

Currently, USA has the highest number of centenarians, followed by Japan, China, India, and Italy. Japan and Italy have the highest proportion of centenarians to the total population. By 2050, China is expected to have the largest centenarian population, followed by Japan, USA, Italy, and India (**Table 2**).

Country	Last Reported Number (Year)	Expected Number by 2050
World	**573,000 (2020)**	**3,676,000**
USA	97,000 (2020)	378,000
Japan	80,000 (2020)	441,000
China	48,000 (2015)	620,000
India	27,000 (2015)	207,000
Italy	25,000 (2015)	216,000

Table 2.
Number of centenarians worldwide and in top five countries (United Nations and national sources).

The oldest supercentenarian with well-documented age was Jeanne Louise Calment (1875–1997) from Arles, France who lived 122 years (**Figure 11**). She married at the age of 21 years, had one pregnancy (gave birth to a girl), and never worked. With the exception of migraines and bilateral cataracts, she was quite healthy and remained mentally sharp until the end of her life. She did daily gymnastics and was socially active. She never took any medication apart from aspirin for migraines. She enjoyed chocolate, drank a small daily amount of wine, smoke a cigarette after each meal, and took a nap in the afternoon. She also had a good sense of humor. To the question "Why do you live so long?", she replied "Because God has forgotten me".

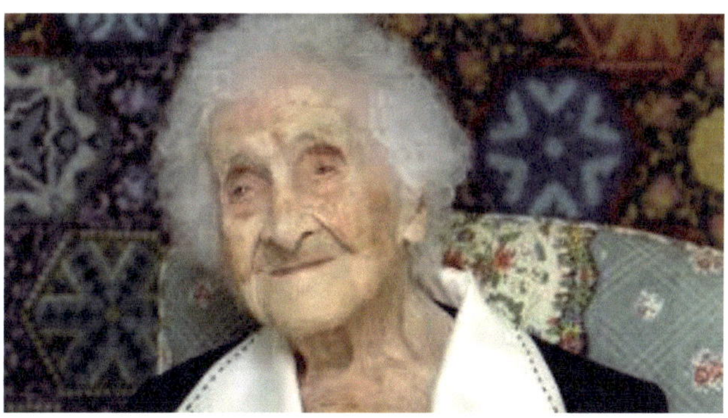

Figure 11.
Jeanne Louise Calment from Arles, France (1875–1997), the oldest confirmed supercentenarian who lived 122 years (Picture downloaded from the internet "Google Images").

3.2 Physiological profile

Maintenance of a proper autophagic activity may contribute to extended longevity. Healthy centenarians have autophagy augmentation as reflected by increased levels of beclin-1, a key regulator of autophagy [57].

Lower thyroid hormone levels and higher TSH levels have been reported to be associated with increased longevity [31, 39, 45–47]. Centenarians have higher TSH levels compared to controls, partly due to a genetic background [31].

Adiponectin levels are elevated in centenarians and associated with a favorable metabolic phenotype. They may contribute to extended longevity [41, 54].

Frailty plays an important role in health outcomes and mortality. A study of Chinese centenarians demonstrated that centenarians are frailer than younger elders. Management of frailty can help achieving healthy longevity [58]. A study of centenarians living in New York City (USA) showed that despite reduced levels of physical functioning and social resources, centenarians were in good mental health suggesting high resilience and ability to adapt to age-associated challenges [59].

3.3 Genetic/epigenetic profile

There is a strong genetic influence in subjects with extreme longevity (**Figure 12**) [3, 8, 10, 27, 31]. Genetic component may include several genetic modifiers each with modest effects, but as a group, they can have a strong impact [27]. Several genotypes known to influence longevity are enriched in centenarians (e.g., *CETP-VV* and *FOXO3A-T*) [10]. Homozygosity in the 405*VV* variant of *CETP* (cholesterol ester transfer protein) gene is associated with lower concentrations of CETP, higher concentrations of high-density lipoprotein (HDL) cholesterol, and larger HDL particle size, all associated with protection against ischemic heart disease and Alzheimer disease. *FOXO3A* (forkhead box O3A) gene is a member of a family of transcription factors mediating insulin action and stress resistance. Several gene mutations responsible of extended longevity are components of endocrine-signaling pathways. For example, centenarians have a variety of genetic alterations in the GH/IGF-1 pathway causing reduced function of GH/IGF-1 pathway that is associated with protection from aging.

Epigenetic processes might also play a role in extreme longevity [8, 9, 11, 26, 30].

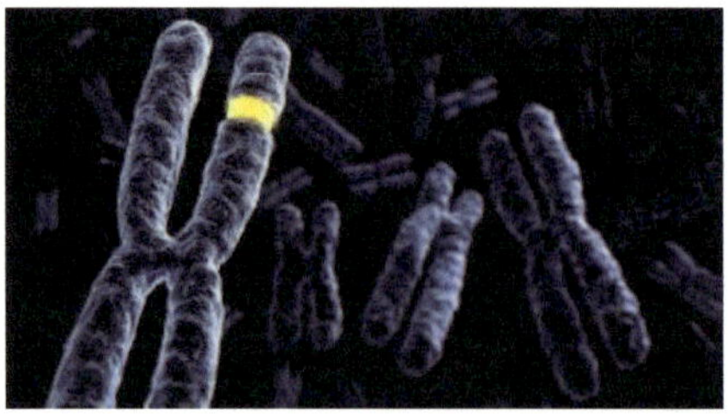

Figure 12.
Several longevity genes are enriched in centenarians (Picture downloaded from the internet "Google Images").

3.4 Lifestyle and environmental characteristics

Lifestyle is an important signature of healthy aging and extreme longevity [26]. There are significant lifestyle (e.g., diet) and cultural (e.g., social life) differences between the native of the top five countries (e.g., USA, Japan, China, India, and Italy) that have the highest numbers of centenarians. However, centenarians share similarities for several lifestyle characteristics (**Figure 13**). The global calorie ingestion is reduced in centenarians in comparison to younger elders. Most centenarians have a plant-based diet, rich in vegetables, fruits, and oils, and usually a restricted intake of dairy products, red meat, and poultry [60]. A study of lifestyle of centenarians living in Zhejiang Province (China) showed significantly higher consumption of fruits, coarse cereals, and pasta, and lower percentage of smoking and engagement in daily recreational activities (watching television, listening to radio) compared to non-centenarians [61].

Additional important lifestyle and environmental characteristics of centenarians are the presence of physical and mental activities (with daily objectives), psychological resilience, optimism, flexibility, and life in small towns with little pollution and significant social relationships. A study of health and functional status of Japanese centenarians suggested that maintenance of physical independence is a key factor of survival into extreme old age [62].

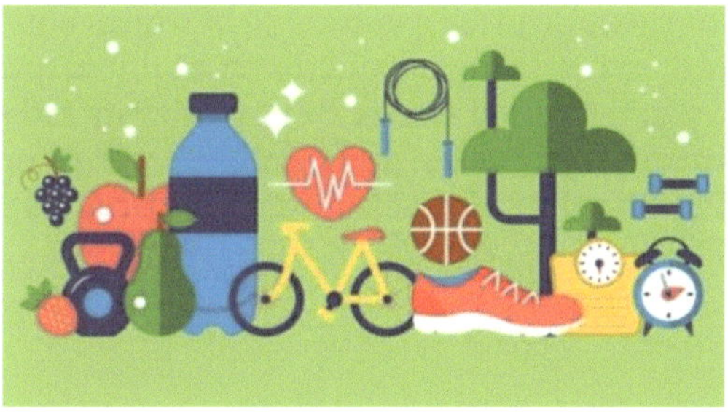

Figure 13.
Centenarians have several common lifestyle characteristics (Picture downloaded from the internet "Google Images").

3.5 Disease occurrence and mortality

Centenarians have variable clinical conditions. Some may have multimorbidity while others have no significant diseases. However, some of the "healthy" centenarians have signs of advanced aging (e.g., visual disorder, hearing loss, and limited locomotor capacity). Centenarian men tend to have better cognitive and physical functional status than centenarian women [3].

Most centenarians have managed to avoid ("escapers"), postpone, or overcome ("survivors") the important age-related and life-threatening diseases and disabilities (e.g., ischemic heart disease, stroke, chronic obstructive pulmonary disease, cancer, respiratory infection, type 2 diabetes, osteoporosis, and dementia) [3, 5, 6]. Supercentenarians can compress morbidity and disability to the very ends of their lives.

A study assessing the place and cause of death of centenarians in England showed that centenarians more likely die of old age/frailty and respiratory infection and less likely of ischemic heart disease and cancer compared to younger elders [4]. Centenarians are relatively protected from cancers (lower incidence, lower metastatic rate, lower mortality). It has been hypothesized that the tumor suppressor gene p53 is a key element in protecting centenarians from cancers [6]. In Spanish centenarians, the likelihood of having the wild-type genotype of *GSTT1*, which is associated with lower cancer risk, was found to be higher than control, young subjects [63]. The top cancers in centenarians are breast, colorectal, prostate, and lung cancers [64].

The main causes of mortality in centenarians compared to younger elders are reported in **Table 3**.

Condition	Mortality Rate	
	Younger Elders	Centenarians
Old age/frailty	1%	28%
Respiratory infection	6%	18%
Ischemic heart disease	19%	9%
Cancer	25%	4%

Table 3.
Main causes of mortality in centenarians compared to younger elders.

4. Interventions to extend longevity

In the absence of the genetic predisposition to become centenarian, there are several potential ways to extend longevity and eventually surpass 100 years. The potential tools that can be proposed to extend longevity include lifestyle, reduction of several life-threatening diseases and disabilities, hormonal replacement or blockade, antioxidants, autophagy inducers, senolytic drugs, stem cell therapy, and gene therapy [8–24, 26, 33–35, 39, 41, 42, 51, 53, 65, 66].

4.1 Lifestyle

Diet rich in vegetables, fruits, fibers, and poor in saturated fat and red meat, even if associated with sarcopenia, may extend longevity [26, 65]. Anti-inflammatory diets like Mediterranean diet are associated with reduced mortality from cardiovascular disease. Drinks containing sugar and alcohol consumption should be limited, and smoking avoided.

Based on animal data, it has been proposed that even in normal weight individuals, caloric restriction (cutting approximately 500 calories/day) without causing malnutrition and subsequent sarcopenia and osteopenia may improve health and extend longevity [8–11, 21, 26, 33, 35, 39, 66]. However, long-term prospective studies in humans are needed to confirm the benefits of this approach. Hypocaloric diet should be implemented in case of overweight or obesity.

Regular exercise can add few more years to life expectancy. Physical fitness is an important predictor of mortality and being able to live an independent life at old age. Potentiation of physical fitness is a valuable anti-aging therapy [11, 51].

In addition, living in a clean and stress-free environment, being mentally active with positive attitude, having daily objectives, and involved in social interactions further contribute to extended longevity.

4.2 Reduction of life-threatening diseases and disabilities

Overweight and obesity should be prevented or managed with appropriate tools (e.g., diet, exercise, drugs, medical devices, and surgery) to decrease comorbidities and mortality [33, 34, 41].

Reduction of other life-threatening diseases and disabilities that can affect longevity (e.g., ischemic heart disease, stroke, chronic obstructive pulmonary disease, cancer, respiratory infection, type 2 diabetes, osteoporosis, and dementia) with lifestyle, drugs, and surgery can improve the quality of life and extend longevity [14, 15, 42].

4.3 Hormonal replacement or blockade

Considering that some hormonal changes during aging are beneficial while others are harmful, it is tempting to use hormonal replacement or blockade to extend longevity [12, 13, 53].

GH represents an interesting and intriguing example in this regard. Although GH promotes health and vitality in young subjects and it is well established that its levels decrease with aging, several studies suggest that reduced GH can be more beneficial for overall health and longevity than excess GH [37, 38, 52]. This discourages the use of GH as an anti-aging treatment. However, additional clinical studies are needed for a definitive conclusion on the role of GH/IGF-1 axis in aging [10].

E replacement therapy in post-menopausal women younger than 60 years has been reported to reduce mortality (extension of longevity) [13].

Treatment with DHEA has beneficial effects on insulin sensitivity (increase) and inflammatory adipokines (decrease) [53]. This can potentially reduce morbidity and mortality.

4.4 Antioxidants

Free radical theory is an important theory of aging [7]. Oxidative stress significantly influence the aging process and longevity. The use of antioxidants to combat aging has received considerable interest [16]. Several antioxidants (e.g., resveratrol and curcumin) are currently under investigation.

4.5 Autophagy inducers

Defects in autophagy have been linked to several diseases that can impact aging and lifespan. Maintenance of a proper autophagic activity with autophagy inducers has the potential to extent longevity [16, 20, 21]. Autophagy inducers include non-pharmacologic tools (e.g., caloric restriction and exercise) and several nutritional supplements and approved drugs (e.g., vitamin D, resveratrol, metformin, and rapamycin) (non-exhaustive list). Novel and more specific autophagy-inducing drugs are under investigation.

4.6 Senolytic drugs

Senescence is a common feature occurring in several tissues and organs during the aging process. Senotherapy represents a promising new therapeutic area [16, 19, 22, 23]. Senolytics are a class of drugs (e.g., dasatinib, quercetin, fisetin, and navitoclax) that selectively clear senescent cells. Several clinical studies are currently planned or ongoing. Results from early pilot studies suggest that senolytic drugs can decrease senescent cells, reduce inflammation, and alleviate frailty.

4.7 Stem cell therapy

Stem cell therapy represents a new emerging era in medicine (**Figure 14**) [16–18]. It has the potential to delay the aging process and, therefore, extend longevity, by better treating chronic diseases and degenerative conditions that impact lifespan.

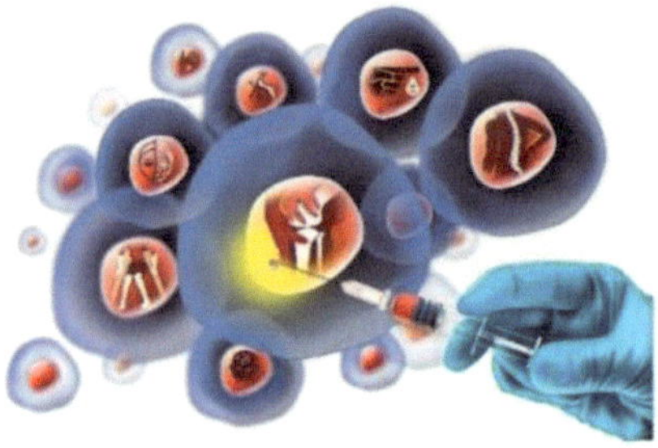

Figure 14.
Stem cell therapy has the potential to delay the aging process and extend longevity (Picture downloaded from the internet "Google Images").

4.8 Gene therapy

Genes are promising research targets to delay the aging process and extend longevity (**Figure 15**) [24]. Gene therapy allows the modulation of the genome architecture using both direct (by gene editing) and indirect (by viral or non-viral vectors) approaches. However, these genetic interventions may be difficult to implement in humans without knowing all the potential health consequences during an entire life.

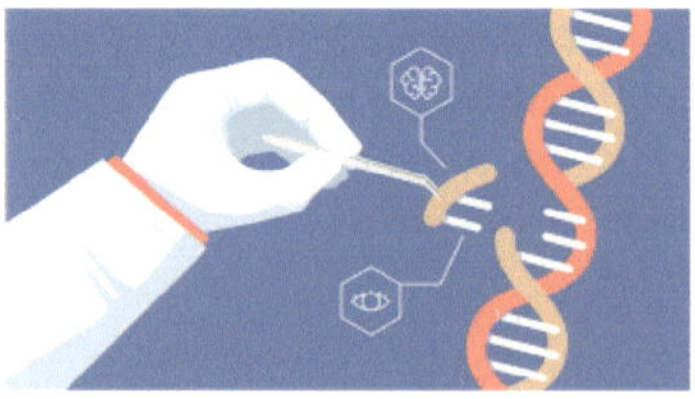

Figure 15.
Genes can be targeted to delay the aging process and extend longevity (Picture downloaded from the internet "Google Images").

5. Consequences of extended longevity

Over the past three decades, the number of very old individuals, especially centenarians, has increased significantly. This has created (and will continue to create) challenges at the individual, family, and societal levels.

5.1 Individual aspects

With the availability of many extra years to live and if health permits, subjects may want to delay retirement age, continue education, undertake a new career, or pursue a passion (**Figure 16**).

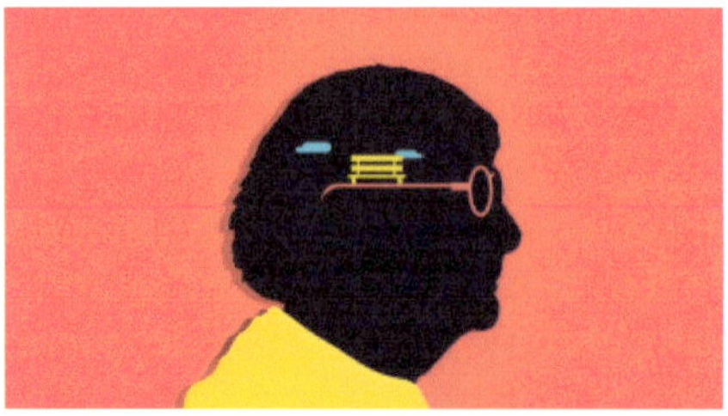

Figure 16.
Healthy elderly can benefit from additional education and job opportunities (Picture downloaded from the internet "Google Images").

5.2 Family aspects

Some centenarians have extended family over multiple generations. These individuals can enjoy interactions with their children, grandchildren, and great-grandchildren at different stages of their life (**Figure 17**).

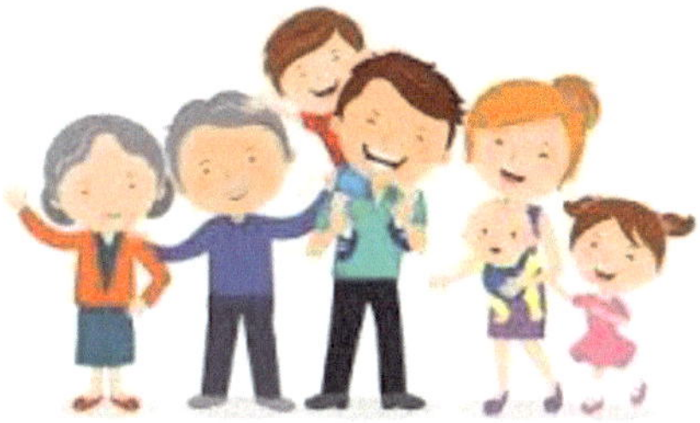

Figure 17.
Centenarians can enjoy multigenerational family interactions (Picture downloaded from the internet "Google Images").

5.3 Societal aspects

There is an urgent need to assess the key characteristics of very old individuals, especially centenarians, across countries to better serve these populations and ensure a high quality of life in their remaining years [1, 2]. There is a requirement for nursing care at home or hospital. Increasing care home bed capacity could reduce dependence on hospital care at the end of life [4, 59].

The payment of pension and social security benefits to a growing number of very old subjects for several decades is a heavy financial challenge for any society. With extended longevity, there is an increasing number of subjects treated for at least three different diseases with at least three different treatments [15]. This will have a significant financial impact for the society (**Figure 18**). However, this situation may not be applicable to all centenarians since some have managed to avoid, postpone, or overcome several important age-related diseases and disabilities.

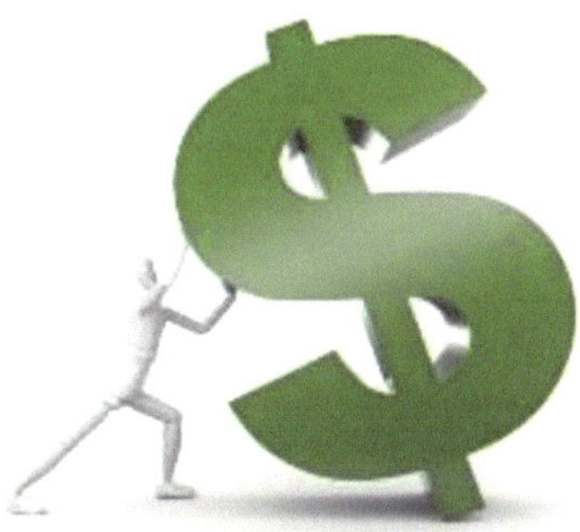

Figure 18.
Centenarians expose societies to financial challenges (Picture downloaded from the internet "Google Images").

6. Conclusions

Long life is a topic of great interest in medicine and among the general public. The increase in life expectancy has led the very old to become the fastest growing segment of the population in several countries.

Centenarians are subjects living 100 years or older. The majority of centenarians are females and a very small fraction of centenarians are supercentenarians.

Most centenarians have managed to avoid, postpone, or overcome the important age-related and life-threatening diseases (e.g., ischemic heart disease, stroke, chronic obstructive pulmonary disease, cancer, respiratory infection, type 2 diabetes, osteoporosis, and dementia).

The continuous increase of the number of centenarians has worldwide practical implications including profound impact on intergenerational interactions and significant financial challenges for any society, especially in relation to medical expenses.

Conflict of interest

The author declares no conflict of interest.

Dedication

The author is dedicating this chapter to his paternal great-grandfather, Abdolrahim Heshmat (1841–1951), a supercentenarian from Shiraz, Iran who lived 110 years.

Author details

Hassan M. Heshmati
Endocrinology Metabolism Consulting, LLC, Anthem, AZ, USA

*Address all correspondence to: hassanheshmati@yahoo.com

References

[1] Jopp DS, Boerner K, Ribeiro O, Rott C. Life at age 100: An international research agenda for centenarian studies. Journal of Aging & Social Policy. 2016;**28**:133-147. DOI: 10.1080/08959420.2016.1161693

[2] He Y, Zhao Y, Yao Y, et al. Cohort profile: The China Hainan Centenarian Cohort Study (CHCCS). International Journal of Epidemiology. 2018;**47**:694-695h. DOI: 10.1039/ije/dyy017

[3] Borras C, Ingles M, Mas-Bargues C, et al. Centenarians: An excellent example of resilience for successful ageing. Mechanisms of Ageing and Development. 2020;**186**:111199. DOI: 10.1016/j.mad.2019.111199

[4] Evans CJ, Ho Y, Daveson BA, Hall S, Higginson IJ, Gao W, on behalf of the GUIDE_Care project. Place and cause of death in centenarians: A population-based observational study in England, 2001 to 2010. PLOS Medicine. 2014;**11**:e1001653. DOI: 10.1371/journal.pmed.1001653

[5] Andersen SL, Sebastiani P, Dworkis DA, Feldman L, Perls TT. Health span approximates life span among many supercentenarians: Compression of morbidity at the approximate limit of life span. The Journals of Gerontology, Series A: Biological Sciences and Medical Sciences. 2012;**67A**:395-405. DOI: 10.1093/gerona/glr223

[6] Salvioli S, Capri M, Bucci L, et al. Why do centenarians escape or postpone cancer? The role of IGF-1, inflammation and p53. Cancer Immunology, Immunotherapy. 2009;**58**:1909-1917. DOI: 10.1007/s00262-008-0639-6

[7] Harman D. Aging: Origin and evolution of the free radical theory of aging: A brief personal history, 1954-2009. Biogerontology. 2009;**10**:773-781. DOI: 10.1007/s10522-009-9234-2

[8] Govindaraju D, Atzmon G, Barzilai N. Genetics, lifestyle and longevity: Lessons from centenarians. Applied & Translational Genomics. 2015;**4**:23-32. DOI: 10.1016/j.atg.2015.01.001

[9] Sgarbieri VC, Pacheco MTB. Healthy human aging: Intrinsic and environmental factors. Brazilian Journal of Food Technology. 2017;**20**:e2017007. DOI: 10.1590/1981-6723.00717

[10] Barzilai N, Huffman DM, Muzumdar RH, Bartke A. The critical role of metabolic pathways in aging. Diabetes. 2012;**61**:1315-1322. DOI: 10.2337/db11-1300

[11] López-Otín C, Galluzzi L, Freije JMP, Madeo F, Kroemer G. Metabolic control of longevity. Cell. 2016;**166**:802-821. DOI: 10.1016/j.cell.2016.07.031

[12] Diamanti-Kandarakis E, Dattilo M, Macut D, et al. Aging and anti-aging: A combo-endocrinology overview. European Journal of Endocrinology. 2017;**176**:R283-R308. DOI: 10.1530/EJE-16-1061

[13] Salpeter SR, Cheng J, Thabane L, Buckley NS, Salpeter EE. Bayesian meta-analysis of hormone therapy and mortality in younger postmenopausal women. The American Journal of Medicine. 2009;**122**:1016-1022. DOI: 10.1016/j.amjmed.2009.05.021

[14] Longo M, Bellastella G, Maiorino MI, Meier JJ, Esposito K, Giugliano D. Diabetes and aging: From treatment goals to pharmacologic therapy. Frontiers in Endocrinology. 2019;**10**:45. DOI: 10.3389/fendo.2019.00045

[15] Barzilai N, Cuervo AM, Austad S. Aging as a biological target for prevention and therapy. Journal of the American Medical Association. DOI: 10.1001/jama.2018.9562

[16] Shetty AK, Kodali M, Upadhya R, Madhu LN. Emerging anti-aging strategies – Scientific basis and efficacy. Aging and Disease. 2018:**9**:1165-1184. DOI: 10.14336/AD.2018.1026

[17] Ullah M, Sun Z. Stem cells and anti-aging genes: Double-edged sword-do the same job of life extension. Stem Cell Research & Therapy. 2018;**9**:3. DOI: 10.1186/s13287-017-0746-4

[18] Schulman IH, Balkan W, Hare JM. Mesenchymal stem cell therapy for aging frailty. Frontiers in Nutrition. 2018;**5**:108. DOI: 10.3389/fnut.2018.00108

[19] Tchkonia T, Kirkland JL. Aging, cell senescence, and chronic disease. Emerging therapeutic strategies. Journal of the American Medical Association. DOI: 10.1001/jama.2018.12440

[20] Levine B, Packer M, Codogno P. Development of autophagy inducers in clinical medicine. The Journal of Clinical Investigation. 2015;**125**:14-24. DOI: 10.1172/JCI73938

[21] Barbosa MC, Grosso RA, Fader CM. Hallmarks of aging: An autophagic perspective. Frontiers in Endocrinology. 2019;**9**:790. DOI: 10.3389/fendo.2018.00790

[22] Myrianthopoulos V. The emerging field of senotherapeutic drugs. Future Medicinal Chemistry. 2018;**10**:2369-2372. DOI: 10.4155/fmc-2018-0234

[23] Kirkland JL, Tchkonia T. Senolytic drugs: From discovery to translation. Journal of Internal Medicine. 2020;**288**:518-536. DOI: 1111/joim.13141

[24] Vaiserman A, De Falco E, Koliada A, Maslova O, Balistreri CR. Anti-ageing gene therapy: Not so far away? Ageing Research Reviews. 2019;**56**:100977. DOI: 10.1016/j.arr.2019.100977

[25] Borges RM. Phenotypic plasticity and longevity in plants and animals: Cause and effect? Journal of Biosciences. 2009;**34**:605-611

[26] Puca AA, Spinelli C, Accardi G, Villa F, Caruso C. Centenarians as a model to discover genetic and epigenetic signatures of healthy ageing. Mechanisms of Ageing and Development. 2018;**174**:95-102. DOI: 10.1016/j.mad.2017.10.004

[27] Sebastiani P, Perls TT. The genetics of extreme longevity: Lessons from the New England Centenarian Study. Frontiers in Genetics. 2012;**3**:277. DOI: 10.3389/fgene.2012.00277

[28] Budovsky A, Craig T, Wang J, et al. LongevityMap: A database of human genetic variants associated with longevity. Trends in Genetics. 2013;**29**:559-560. DOI: 10.1016/j.tig.2013.08.003

[29] Shadyab AH, LaCroix AZ. Genetic factors associated with longevity: A review of recent findings. Ageing Research Reviews. 2015;**19**:1-7. DOI: 10.1016/j.arr.2014.10.005

[30] Horvath S, Pirazzini C, Bacalini MG, et al. Decreased epigenetic age of PBMCs from Italian semi-supercentenarians and their offspring. Aging. 2015;**7**:1159-1170

[31] Barzilai N, Gabriely I. Genetic studies reveal the role of the endocrine and metabolic systems in aging. The Journal of Clinical Endocrinology & Metabolism. 2010;**95**:4493-4500. DOI: 10.1210/jc.2010-0859

[32] Bektas A, Schurman SH, Sen R, Ferrucci L. Aging, inflammation and

the environment. Experimental Gerontology. 2018;**105**:10-18. 10.1016/j.exger.2017.12.015

[33] Lorenzini A. How much should we weigh for a long and healthy life span? The need to reconcile caloric restriction versus longevity with body mass index versus mortality data. Frontiers in Endocrinology. 2014;**5**:121. DOI: 10.3389/fendo.2014.00121

[34] The Global BMI Mortality Collaboration. Body-mass index and all-cause mortality: Individual-participant-data meta-analysis of 239 prospective studies in four continents. Lancet. 2016;**388**:776-786. DOI: 10.1016/S0140-6736(16)30175-1

[35] Allard JB, Duan C. Comparative endocrinology of aging and longevity regulation. Frontiers in Endocrinology. 2011;**2**:75. DOI: 10.3389/fendo.2011.00075

[36] Chen TT, Maevsky EI, Uchitel ML. Maintenance of homeostasis in the aging hypothalamus: The central and peripheral roles of succinate. Frontiers in Endocrinology. 2015;**6**:7. DOI: 10.3389/fendo.2015.00007

[37] Colon G, Saccon T, Schneider A, et al. The enigmatic role of growth hormone in age-related diseases, cognition, and longevity. GeroScience. 2019;**41**:759-774. DOI: 10.1007/s11357-019-00096-w

[38] Bartke A. Growth hormone and aging. Reviews in Endocrine and Metabolic Disorders. DOI: 10.1007/s11154-020-09593-2

[39] Bowers J, Terrien J, Clerget-Froidevaux MS, et al. Thyroid hormone signaling and homeostasis during aging. Endocrine Reviews. 2013;**34**:556-589. DOI: 10.1210/er.2012-1056

[40] Araujo AB, Dixon JM, Suarez EA, Hassan Murad M, Guey LT, Wittert GA. Endogenous testosterone and mortality in men: A systematic review and meta-analysis. The Journal of Clinical Endocrinology & Metabolism. 2011;**96**:3007-3019. DOI: 10.1210/jc.2011-1137

[41] Mancuso P, Bouchard B. The impact of aging on adipose function and adipokine synthesis. Frontiers in Endocrinology. 2019;**10**:137. DOI: 10.3389/fendo.2019.00137

[42] Beard JR, Officer A, Araujo de Carvalho I, et al. The World report on ageing and health: A policy framework for healthy ageing. Lancet. 2016;**387**:2145-2154. DOI: 10.1016/S0140-6736(15)00516-4

[43] Olshansky SJ. From lifespan to healthspan. Journal of the American Medical Association. DOI: 10.1001/jama.2018.12621

[44] Wang Y, Hekimi S. Mitochondrial dysfunction and longevity in animals: Untangling the knot. Science. 2015;**350**:1204-1207. DOI: 10.1126/science.aac4357

[45] Peeters RP. Thyroid function and longevity: New insights into an old dilemma. The Journal of Clinical Endocrinology & Metabolism. 2009;**94**:4658-4660. DOI: 10.1210/jc.2009-2198

[46] Atzmon G, Barzilai N, Hollowell JG, Surks MI, Gabriely I. Extreme longevity is associated with increased serum thyrotropin. The Journal of Clinical Endocrinology & Metabolism. 2009;**94**:1251-1254. DOI: 10.1210/jc.2008-2325

[47] Aggarwal N, Razvi S. Thyroid and aging or the aging thyroid? An evidence-based analysis of the literature. Journal of Thyroid Research. DOI: 10.1155/2013/481287

[48] Burger HG, Hale GE, Robertson DM, Dennerstein L.

A review of hormonal changes during the menopausal transition: Focus on findings from the Melbourne Women's Midlife Health Project. Human Reproduction Update. 2007;**13**:559-565. DOI: 10.1093/humupd/dmm020

[49] Orentreich N, Brind JL, Vogelman JH, Andres R, Baldwin H. Long-term longitudinal measurements of plasma dehydroepiandrosterone sulfate in normal men. The Journal of Clinical Endocrinology & Metabolism. 1992;**75**:1002-1004. DOI: 10.1210/jcem.75.4.1400863

[50] Merideth MA, Gordon LB, Clauss S, et al. Phenotype and course of Hutchinson-Gilford progeria syndrome. The New England Journal of Medicine. 2008;**358**:592-604

[51] Castillo-Garzón MJ, Ruiz JR, Ortega FB, Gutiérrez ÁG. Anti-aging therapy through fitness enhancement. Clinical Interventions in Aging. 2006;**1**:213-220

[52] van der Spoel E, Jansen SW, Akintola AA, et al. Growth hormone secretion is diminished and tightly controlled in humans enriched for familial longevity. Aging Cell. 2016;**15**:1126-1131. DOI: 10.1111/acel.12519

[53] Weiss EP, Villareal DT, Fontana L, Han DH, Holloszy JO. Dehydroepiandrosterone (DHEA) replacement decreases insulin resistance and lowers inflammatory cytokines in aging humans. Aging. 2011;**3**:533-542. DOI: 10.18632/aging.100327

[54] Arai Y, Hirose N. Adiponectin and healthy aging in centenarians. Anti-Aging Medicine. 2012;**9**:1-5

[55] Faggiano A, Del Prete M, Marciello F, Marotta V, Ramundo V, Colao A. Thyroid diseases in elderly. Minerva Endocrinologica. 2011;**36**:211-231

[56] GBD 2017 Mortality Collaborators. Global, regional, and national age-sex-specific mortality and life expectancy, 1950-2017: A systematic analysis for the global burden of disease study 2017. Lancet. 2018;**392**:1684-1735

[57] Emanuele E, Minoretti P, Sanchis-Gomar F, et al. Can enhanced autophagy be associated with human longevity? Serum levels of the autophagy biomarker beclin-1 are increased in healthy centenarians. Rejuvenation Research. 2014;**17**:518-524. DOI: 10.1089/rej.2014.1607

[58] Gu D, Feng Q. Frailty still matters to health and survival in centenarians: The case of China. BMC Geriatrics. 2015;**15**:159. DOI: 10.1186/s12877-015-0159-0

[59] Jopp DS, Park MKS, Lehrfeld J, Paggi ME. Physical, cognitive, social and mental health in near-centenarians and centenarians living in New York City: Findings from the Fordham Centenarian Study. BMC Geriatrics. 2016;**16**:1. DOI: 10.1186/s12877-015-0167-0

[60] Davinelli S, Willcox DC, Scapagnini G. Extending healthy ageing: Nutrient sensitive pathway and centenarian population. Immunity & Ageing. 2012;**9**:9. DOI: 10.1186/1742-4933-9-9

[61] Rong C, Shen SH, Xiao LW, et al. A comparative study on the health status and behavioral lifestyle of centenarians and non-centenarians in Zhejiang Province, China – A cross-sectional study. Frontiers in Public Health. 2019;**7**:344. DOI: 10.3389/fpubh.2019.00344

[62] Arai Y, Inagaki H, Takayama M, et al. Physical independence and mortality at the extreme limit of life span: Supercentenarians study in Japan. The Journals of Gerontology, Series A: Biological Sciences and Medical

Sciences. 2014;**69**:486-494. DOI: 10.1093/gerona/glt146

[63] Ruiz JR, Fiuza-Luces C, Buxens A, et al. Are centenarians genetically predisposed to lower disease risk? AGE. 2012;**34**:1269-1283. DOI: 10.1007/s11357-011-9296-3

[64] Joseph SC, Delcastilo E, Osiro S, Loukas M. Common cancers in centenarians. Medical Science Monitor. 2014;**20**:18-23. DOI: 10.12659/MSM.889877

[65] Pereira da Silva A, Valente A, Chaves C, et al. Characterization of Portuguese centenarian eating habits, nutritional biomarkers, and cardiovascular risk: A case control study. Oxidative Medicine and Cellular Longevity. DOI: 10.1155/2018/5296168

[66] Abbasi J. Can a diet that mimics fasting turn back the clock? Journal of the American Medical Association. 2017;**318**:227-229

Chapter 2

A Comprehensive Overview of Mobility and Aging in the Year 2020 (and beyond)

Melissa Lunsman O'Connor

Abstract

Mobility can be defined as the ability to move effectively and purposefully though the environment in order to accomplish goals. Mobility can be conceptualized and measured in four broad ways. First, the speed, success, and quality of specific movements can be measured, such as gait and balance. Second, one can assess a person's ability to complete activities of daily living (ADLs) and instrumental activities of daily living (IADLs) that involve movement. Third, the occurrence of adverse events, such as falls and motor vehicle crashes, can be measured. Finally, the range of a person's movement inside and outside the home can be assessed. Regardless of how it is conceptualized, mobility is one of the most important determinants of quality of life and independence in adulthood. Unfortunately, the prevalence of mobility limitations increases with age. This book chapter will provide a comprehensive overview of mobility among older adults.

Keywords: mobility, aging, older adults, elderly, quality of life

1. Introduction

In broad terms, mobility can be defined as the ability to move effectively and purposefully though the environment in order to accomplish tasks or achieve goals [1]. Mobility is impacted by personal, socio-economic, and environmental factors and, in turn, influences qualify of life, autonomy, independence, and everyday functioning [1, 2]. Verbrugge, Gruber-Baldini, and Fozard [3] characterized mobility as the most important functional domain for older adults, and current research has continued to support that assertion [4, 5]. Unfortunately, the prevalence of mobility limitations increases with age [1, 2]. Thus, mobility is a salient research area. This chapter will provide a comprehensive overview of mobility among older adults, including different aspects of mobility, factors that influence mobility, and future directions for study.

2. Aspects of mobility

Mobility is a broad construct. It can refer to the physical ability to move, or the extent of movement in time and space [6]. Ball and Owsley [7] described four general ways in which mobility can be measured. First, the speed, success, and quality of specific movements can be measured, such as gait and balance. Second, mobility can be assessed by indicators of everyday functioning, including activities of daily living (ADLs), instrumental activities of daily living (IADLs), and driving. Third, mobility can be measured by the occurrence of adverse events, such as falls or motor vehicle crashes. Finally, the range of a person's movement inside and outside the home can be assessed. These four interrelated aspects of mobility, and how they are measured, are summarized below.

2.1 Specific movements

Researchers use many performance-based and self-report measures to quantify physical mobility among older adults. Studies often assess a participant's unassisted walking speed, chair-rise time, ability to maintain different standing positions, and stair climbing ability [7, 8]. Two widely-used performance-based tests are the Turn 360° Test, which assesses the number of steps an examinee takes to turn in a complete circle [9], and the Timed Up and Go Test (TUG), which measures the number of seconds required for an examinee to rise from a chair, walk 3 meters, return to the chair, and resume sitting [10]. There are numerous batteries that incorporate several performance-based tests, such as the Short Physical Performance Battery [11]. Gait mats and body sensors can be used to measure specific components of physical performance, such as gait velocity, stride length, and foot trajectory [12]. Self-report questionnaires are also available for assessing older adults' perceptions of their physical mobility (e.g., [13]).

Physical mobility is often the first area in which older adults experience difficulties. Risk factors for poor physical performance include a sedentary lifestyle, co-morbid diseases, depressive symptoms, and metabolic syndrome [8, 14]. Studies have also found positive relationships between physical mobility and cognitive abilities like memory, attention, and speed of processing [12, 15]. Independent of health and demographic variables, impaired physical mobility is associated with institutionalization, morbidity, mortality, functional disability, and declines in other domains of mobility, including everyday functioning [16, 17].

2.2 Everyday functioning

2.2.1 ADLs and IADLs

ADLs that involve mobility include dressing, toileting, and transferring, and mobility-related IADLs include shopping, cooking, housework, and driving. These everyday tasks are critical for independent living and health maintenance [18]. There are numerous informant-based instruments for assessing ADL and IADL performance, including the Katz Index [19] and the Older Adults Resources Scale [20]. Most of these scales ask respondents (or their proxies) to rate the level of independence at which they can perform different activities, or to provide difficulty ratings for the activities. ADLs and IADLs can also be measured via performance-based tasks, although some tests (e.g., the Timed IADL) are not mobility-oriented [21, 22].

The consideration of ADLs and IADLs places mobility within a larger context. According to the Disablement Process theory [23], ADL and IADL behaviors are socially defined, so impaired performance on these tasks indicates disability as well as reduced functional capacity. Older adults may have reduced physical capabilities but experience little-to-no disability that affects quality of life, partly due to compensatory strategies and the use of assistive technology [24]. When impaired performance on ADLs or IADLs does reach the level of disability, it is linked to institutionalization, increased health care costs, mortality, and falls [25].

Other predictors of ADL/IADL disability include co-morbid diseases, sensory impairments, depressive symptoms, and cognitive decline [26, 27]. Wadley and colleagues [28] examined 5-year changes in self-reported IADL functioning among older adults with mild cognitive impairment (MCI). Participants with MCI showed faster rates of decline than participants without MCI. Performance on cognitively demanding IADLs, such as counting money, is associated with performance on mobility-related IADLs [29]. The ability to utilize transportation is an important mobility-related IADL. In countries without widespread public transportation systems, like the United States, transportation often involves driving. Driving will be given a special focus below, given its importance for many older adults.

2.2.2 Driving

In the United States, O'Neill [30] found that 77% of adults aged 55 or older characterized driving as "very essential" or "essential" for daily life. It is often necessary for maintaining social connections and accessing employment, shopping, entertainment, and health care services. A driver's license also represents autonomy, status, and independence [18, 31]. Thus, older adults tend to maintain their driving status with age. Jette and Branch [32] found that about 75% of older individuals who were self-reliant drivers in 1974 continued to be self-reliant ten years later. Using data from a national longitudinal study, Foley, Heimovitz, Guralnik, and Brock [33] found a driving life expectancy of 11 years for male and female drivers aged 70–74. Even older adults with physical frailty [34] and dementia [35] may continue to drive.

Studies of driving often use self-report measures that assess how often one drives and in what situations one drives [36]. Driving behaviors can also be assessed objectively by on-road tests, simulators, or GPS tracking technology [37, 38]. There are significant positive correlations between self-reported and objectively measured driving patterns [37]. However, respondents tend to underestimate the number of trips they take and to provide inaccurate estimates of their mileage [38, 39].

Studies of objective driving performance have found that older drivers had the most trouble with lane positioning, yielding, merging, and blind spot monitoring [40, 41]. Age-related declines in vision, hearing, physical abilities, health, and cognition can make driving more difficult and riskier for older individuals [42–44]. Older adults often compensate for these deficits by self-regulating their driving, or adjusting their driving to avoid particularly hazardous situations. This may include driving less frequently, restricting distance, driving more slowly, driving with a companion, or avoiding night driving, bad weather, and busy traffic [43, 45–47]. These behaviors can allow older drivers to maintain a desirable level of mobility without compromising safety [48]. Self-reported reasons for restricting driving, and stopping driving altogether, include vision problems, health co-morbidities, depressive symptoms, and lower cognitive performance [44, 49, 50]. Adverse events such as falls and crashes may also lead to restricted driving, and restricted mobility in general [50].

2.3 Adverse events

2.3.1 Falls

Mobility difficulties may be indicated by the occurrence, frequency, and/or severity of adverse events, such as injuries, falls, and motor vehicle crashes. Falls are usually assessed via self-report items that ask how often a respondent fell within the preceding few months/years, whether any falls resulted in injury, and whether particular factors contributed to the falls [44, 51]. Daily calendars can also be used to track falls over time [52].

Each year, about one-third of community-dwelling older adults experience a fall in the United States, and 5–15% of these individuals require medical attention [53, 54]. Seventy percent of all fall-related deaths occur in adults over age 65 [55]. In addition to causing injuries, morbidity, and mortality, falls can have devastating psychological consequences. Fear of falling is associated with loss of confidence and avoidance of physical activities, leading to further functional declines [54].

Falls have both extrinsic (i.e., environmental hazards) and intrinsic precipitating factors [56]. The majority of older adults who fall are indoors and alone at the time [57]. Gait and balance abnormalities are strongly associated with falls, and interventions to improve these abilities can significantly decrease the risk of falls [58, 59]. Other risk factors for falls may include poor vision, medication use, poor health, and cognitive impairment [44, 60, 61]. Vance et al. [44] noted that these same factors are also associated with motor vehicle crashes. Indeed, individuals with a history of falls are also more likely to sustain a motor vehicle crash [62].

2.3.2 Motor vehicle crashes

Studies of older driver safety commonly use crashes as outcome measures, which may be quantified by self-reports or state records. Self-reports are practical and have been found to correlate with on-road driving performance [41]. State records are standardized and objective, but only provide information on crashes reported to the police [63]. Many studies have specifically focused on at-fault crashes (e.g., [62]), crashes resulting in injuries and/or fatalities [64], or state-recorded traffic violations (e.g., [40]).

Some studies have shown that, compared to middle-aged drivers, drivers aged 75 and older have higher crash rates per driver per mile driven [65, 66]. However, older drivers typically drive shorter distances than younger drivers, which may result in exaggerated crash rate estimates, or "low mileage bias" [67, 68]. Despite this, older drivers have a greater risk of dying or sustaining serious injuries in a crash because of their increased fragility (e.g., [64, 65]). Compared to young and middle-aged drivers, older drivers are also more likely to experience multi-vehicle crashes at intersections, are more often considered at-fault, and may be more likely to injure other road users [66, 69, 70].

Risk factors for crashes include age-related declines in physical abilities, health, vision, and cognitive abilities (e.g., [48, 62]), as well as previous accidents [71]. Visual attention and speed of processing are particularly important for safe driving [48, 72]. For example, the Useful Field of View Test (UFOV), a computerized speed of processing and visual attention measure, can predict crash involvement as well as other driving outcomes (e.g., [72–74]).

2.4 Spatial mobility

Measures of physical movements, ADLs/IADLs, and adverse events like crashes fail to consider an important aspect of mobility—the extent of one's movement within the environment. Spatial mobility can be characterized by the concept of life space. The term "life space" was first proposed by May, Nayak, and Isaacs [75], who defined it as a series of zones ranging from the bedroom to outside the home. According to Parker, Baker, and Allman [76], life space captures person-environment interactions that other measures of mobility do not.

Stalvey and colleagues [51] developed a commonly used, self-report measure of life space, the Life Space Questionnaire (LSQ). The LSQ measures how far a respondent traveled from home in the weeks and months prior to the assessment, and it is reliable and validated for use with older adults. A similar questionnaire is the Life-Space Assessment, which measures the extent, frequency, and independence of a person's mobility [77]. Life space can also be measured via modern tracking technologies [78].

Studies have found that most older adults travel regularly outside their towns, but 11–34% of older adults have life space confined to their homes [79, 80]. Using a modified version of the LSQ, Lochner and colleagues [80] found that 12% of Caucasians and 22% of African Americans had life space limited to their bedroom. Restricted life space is associated with social isolation, cognitive impairment, visual impairment, fear of falling, and impairments in other aspects of mobility, including gait speed [81–84]. Restrictions in life space have been found to precede impairments in IADL performance [77].

It is clear that, while the different aspects of mobility may be regarded as distinct variables, they are interconnected in complex ways. They all predict quality of life and independence, and there are common risk factors for reductions in mobility. The topic of safe mobility for older adults will become increasingly salient over the next few decades as the older population grows. Currently, the pool of literature on mobility and aging is large and growing. However, there are still a number of areas that merit further exploration. Some potential future directions are summarized below.

3. Future directions

First, future research on mobility and aging should include more samples from underrepresented groups. Research involving minority groups and developing countries is lacking. In addition, studies have tended to focus on healthy, community-dwelling older adults. More research with clinically impaired populations should be conducted, especially with regard to interventions.

Second, several large-scale longitudinal studies have been conducted with mobility-related variables and multiple waves of data. More studies should use these data to test complex models, such as structural equation models with mediators and moderators, or time-varying relationships between variables. It is likely that declines in cognition, health, and other variables precede restrictions in mobility, which in turn exacerbates the previous declines. Cohort effects on mobility should also be examined, because this may account for cross-sectional differences between age groups, as well as gender differences.

Third, researchers should continue utilizing technology to obtain objective measurements of mobility. This should steadily become more feasible, as technology becomes more affordable and user-friendly. With regard to driving and life space, for example, data from tracking devices can be combined with self-report assessments to yield a comprehensive picture.

Finally, research on interventions that can preserve mobility in older age is increasingly important. Promising interventions include fall prevention programs, assistive devices, and cognitive training programs. There are numerous products and services being marketed to older adults, but not all of them have been tested scientifically. Additionally, it is important to know which interventions are the most effective.

4. Conclusions

Mobility is a broad construct that can be defined and quantified in many ways. Whether it is measured in terms of physical movements, the ability to carry out

ADLs and IADLs, adverse events, or life space, the loss of mobility negatively affects autonomy, health, and quality of life. Mobility is a particularly salient issue for older adults, because age-related declines in sensory, cognitive, and physical abilities are risk factors for mobility limitations.

Author details

Melissa Lunsman O'Connor
North Dakota State University, Fargo, ND, USA

*Address all correspondence to: melissa.oconnor@ndsu.edu

References

[1] Webber, S.C., M.M. Porter, and V.H. Menec, Mobility in older adults: A comprehensive framework. The Gerontologist, 2010. 50(4): p. 443-450.

[2] Dickerson, A.E., et al., Transportation and Aging: An Updated Research Agenda to Advance Safe Mobility among Older Adults Transitioning from Driving to Non-driving. The Gerontologist, 2019. 59(2): p. 215-221.

[3] Verbrugge, L., A. Gruber-Baldini, and J. Fozard, Age differences and age changes in activities: Baltimore longitudinal study of aging. The Journals of Gerontology. Series B, Psychological and Social Sciences., 1996. 51(1): p. 30-41.

[4] Mulry, C., et al., The relationship between community mobility, health status, and quality of life (QOL) in older adults. American Journal of Occupational Therapy, 2019. 73: p. 7311505078.

[5] McInnes, L., et al., Mobility in community dwelling older adults: Predicting successful mobility using an instrumented battery of novel measures. The Journal of Frailty and Aging, 2020. 9: p. 68-73.

[6] Ball, K.K. and C. Owsley, Increasing mobility and reducing accidents of older drivers, in Mobilty and transportation in the elderly, K.W. Schaie and M. Pietrucha, Editors. 2000, Springer: New York. p. 213-250.

[7] Lee, J.S., et al., Weight change, weight change intention, and the incidence of mobility limitation in well-functioning community-dwelling older adults. Journals of Gerontology. Series A, Biological Sciences and Medical Sciences, 2005. 60(8): p. 1007-1012.

[8] Patel, K.V., et al., Midlife physical activity and mobility in older age: The InCHANTI study. American Journal of Preventative Medicine, 2006. 31(3): p. 217-224.

[9] Steinhagen-Thiessen, E. and M. Borchelt, Morbidity, medication, and functional limitations in very old age, in The Berlin Aging Study: Aging from 70 to 100, P.B. Baltes and K.U. Mayer, Editors. 1999, Cambridge University Press: New York. p. 131-166.

[10] Podsiadlo, D. and S. Richardson, The Timed Up & Go: A test of basic functional mobility for frail elderly persons. Journal of the American Geriatrics Society, 1991(39): p. 141-148.

[11] Ostir, G.V., et al., Reliability and sensitivity to change assessed for a summary measure of lower body function: Results from the Women's Health and Aging Study. Journal of Clinical Epidemiology, 2002. 55: p. 916-921.

[12] Holtzer, R., et al., Cognitive processes related to gait velocity: Results from the Einstein Aging Study. Neuropsychology, 2006. 20(2): p. 215-223.

[13] Shumway-Cook, A., et al., Assessing environmentally determined mobility disability: Self-report versus observed community mobility. Journal of the American Geriatrics Society, 2005. 53: p. 700-704.

[14] Blazer, D.G., C.F. Hybels, and G.G. Fillenbaum, Metabolic syndrome predicts mobility decline in a community-based sample of older adults. Journal of the American Geriatrics Society, 2006. 54: p. 502-506.

[15] Kimura, N., et al., Memory and physical activity in physically and cognitively-independent elderly people. Geriatrics and Gerontology International, 2007. 7: p. 258-265.

[16] Boyle, P.A., et al., Physical activity is associated with incident disability in community-based older persons. Journal of the American Geriatrics Society, 2007. 55: p. 195-201.

[17] Rolland, Y., et al., Physical performance measures as predictors of mortality in a cohort of community-dwelling older French women. European Journal of Epidemiology, 2006. 21: p. 113-122.

[18] Barr, R.A., More road to travel by: Implications for mobility and safety in late life. Gerotechnology, 2002. 2(1): p. 50-24.

[19] Katz, S., et al., The index of ADL: A standardized measure of biological and psychosocial function. Journal of the American Geriatrics Society, 1963. 31: p. 721-727.

[20] Fillenbaum, G.G. and M.A. Smyer, The development, validity and reliability of the OARS multidimensional functional assessment questionnaire. Journal of Gerontology, 1981(36): p. 428-434.

[21] Owsley, C., et al., Timed instrumental activities of daily living tasks: Relationship to visual function in older adults. Optometry and Vision Science, 2001. 78(5): p. 350-359.

[22] McDougall, G.J., et al., Predictors of instrumental activities of daily living in community-dwelling older adults. Archives of Psychiatric Nursing, 2019. 33(5): p. 43-50.

[23] Verbrugge, L.M. and A.M. Jette, The disablement process. Social Science and Medicine, 1994. 31(1): p. 1-14.

[24] Roelands, M., et al., Awareness among community-dwelling elderly of assistive devices for mobility and self-care and attitudes towards their use. Social Science and Medicine, 2002. 54: p. 1441-1451.

[25] Schupf, N., et al., Decline in cognitive and functional skills increases mortality risk in nondemented elderly. Neurology, 2005. 65: p. 1218-1226.

[26] Whitson, H.E., et al., The combined effect of visual impairment and cognitive impairment on disability in older people. Journal of the American Geriatrics Society, 2007. 55(885-891).

[27] Wood, K.M., et al., Sensory and cognitive factors influencing functional ability in older adults. Gerontology, 2005. 51: p. 131-141.

[28] Wadley, V.G., et al., Changes in everyday function among individuals with psychometrically defined mild cognitive impairment. Journal of the American Geriatrics Society, 2007. 55(8): p. 1192-1198.

[29] Ackerman, M.L., et al., Examination of cognitive and instrumental functional performance as indicators for driving cessation risk across 3 years. The Gerontologist, 2008. 48(6): p. 802-810.

[30] O'Neill, D., Safe mobility for older people. Reviews in Clinical Gerontology, 2000. 10: p. 181-191.

[31] Shope, J.T., What does giving up driving mean to older drivers and why is it so difficult? Generations, 2003. 2: p. 57-59.

[32] Jette, A.M. and L.G. Branch, A ten-year follow-up of driving patterns among the community-dwelling elderly. Human Factors, 1992. 34(1): p. 25-31.

[33] Foley, D.J., et al., Driving life expectancy of persons aged 70 years and older in the United States. American Journal of Public Health and the Nations Health, 2002. 92(8): p. 1284-1289.

[34] Carr, D.B., et al., Characteristics of frail older adult drivers. Journal of the American Geriatrics Society, 2006. 54: p. 1125-1129.

[35] Croston, J., et al., Driving retirement in older adults with dementia. Topics in Geriatric Rehabilitation, 2009. 25(2): p. 154-162.

[36] Owsley, C., et al., Older drivers and cataract: Driving habits and crash risk. The Journals of Gerontology. Series A, Biological and Medical Sciences, 1999. 54: p. 203-211.

[37] Marshall, S.C., et al., Measurement of driving patterns of older adults using data logging devices with and without global positioning system capability. Traffic Injury Prevention, 2007. 8(3): p. 260-266.

[38] Blanchard, R.A., A.M. Myers, and M.M. Porter, Correspondence between self-reported and objective measures of driving exposure and patterns in older drivers. Accident Analysis and Prevention, 2010. 42: p. 523-529.

[39] Staplin, L., K.W. Gish, and J.J. Joyce, Low mileage bias and related policy implications - a cautionary note. Accident Analysis and Prevention, 2008. 40: p. 1249-1252.

[40] Classen, S., et al., Traffic violations versus driving errors of older adults: Informing clinical practice. American Journal of Occupational Therapy, 2010. 64(2): p. 233-241.

[41] Wood, J.M., et al., The on-road difficulties of older drivers and their relationship with self-reported motor vehicle crashes. Journal of the American Geriatrics Society, 2009. 57(11): p. 2062-2069.

[42] Turano, K.A., et al., Poor sense of direction is associated with constricted driving space in older drivers. Journals of Gerontology. Series B, Psychological Sciences and Social Sciences, 2009. 64(3): p. 348-355.

[43] Unsworth, C.A., et al., To continue, modify or relinquish driving: Findings from a longitudinal study of healthy aging. Gerontology, 2007. 53(6): p. 423-431.

[44] Vance, D.E., et al., Predictors of driving exposure and avoidance in a field study of older drivers from the state of Maryland. Accident Analysis and Prevention, 2006. 38: p. 823-831.

[45] Kostyniuk, L.P. and L.J. Molnar, Self-regulatory driving practices among older adults: Health, age, and sex effects. Accident Analysis and Prevention, 2008. 40(4): p. 1576-1580.

[46] Donorfio, L.K., et al., To drive or not to drive, that isn't the question - the meaning of self-regulation among older drivers. Journal of Safety Research, 2009. 40(3): p. 221-226.

[47] Charlton, J.L., et al., Characteristics of older drivers who adopt self-regulatory driving behaviours. Transportation Research Part F, 2006. 9: p. 363-373.

[48] Anstey, K.J., et al., Cognitive, sensory, and physical factors enabling driving safety in older adults. Clinical Psychology Review, 2005. 25: p. 45-65.

[49] West, C.G., et al., Vision and driving self-restriction in older adults. Journal of the American Geriatrics Society, 2003. 51: p. 1348-1355.

[50] Ang, B.H., et al., To reduce or to cease: A systematic review and meta-analysis of quantitative studies on self-regulation of driving. Journal of Safety Research, 2019. 70: p. 243-251.

[51] Stalvey, B.T., et al., The Life Space Questionnaire: A measure of the extent of mobility of older adults. Journal of Applied Gerontology, 1999. 18(4): p. 460-478.

[52] Hannan, M.T., et al., Optimizing the tracking of falls in studies of

older participants: Comparision of quarterly telephone recall with monthly falls calendars in the MOBILIZE Boston Study. American Journal of Epidemiology, 2010. 171(9): p. 1031-1036.

[53] Akyol, A.D., Falls in the elderly: What can be done? International Nursing Review, 2007. 54: p. 191-196.

[54] Ganz, D.A. and N.K. Latham, Prevention of Falls in Community-Dwelling Older Adults. New England Journal of Medicine, 2020. 382: p. 734-743.

[55] Edelberg, H.K., How to prevent falls and injuries in patients with impaired mobility. Geriatrics, 2001. 56(3): p. 41-45.

[56] Morley, J.E., Falls – where do we stand? Missouri Medicine, 2007. 104(1): p. 63-67.

[57] Roe, B., et al., Older people and falls: Health status, quality of life, care networks, prevention and views on service use following a recent fall. Journal of Clinical Nursing, 2009. 18(16): p. 2261-2272.

[58] Muir, S.W., et al., Balance impairment as a risk factor for falls in community-dwelling older adults who are high-functioning: A prospective study. Physical Therapy, 2010. 90(3): p. 338-347.

[59] Pfortmueller, C.A., G. Lindner, and A.K. Exadaktylos, Reducing fall risk in the elderly: Risk factors and fall prevention, a systematic review. Minerva Medica, 2014. 105(4): p. 275-281.

[60] Faulkner, K.A., et al., Lifestyle predicts falls independent of physical risk factors. Osteoporosis International, 2009. 20(12): p. 2025-2034.

[61] Enderlin, C., et al., Summary of factors contributing to falls in older adults and nursing implications. Geriatric Nursing, 2015. 36(5): p. 397-406.

[62] Cross, J.M., et al., Visual and medical risk factors for motor vehicle collison involvement among older drivers. British Journal of Ophthalmology, 2009. 93(3): p. 400-404.

[63] Owsley, C., Clinical and research issues on older drivers: Future directions. Alzheimer Disease and Associated Disorders, 1997. 11(Suppl. 1): p. 3-7.

[64] Hanrahan, R.B., et al., The association of driver age with traffic injury severity in Wisconsin. Traffic Injury Prevention, 2009. 10(4): p. 361-370.

[65] Eberhard, J., Older drivers' "high per-mile crash involvement": The implications for licensing authorities. Traffic Injury Prevention, 2008. 9(4): p. 284-290.

[66] McGwin, G.J., Jr. and D.B. Brown, Characteristics of traffic crashes among young, middle-aged, and older drivers. Accident Analysis and Prevention, 1999. 31: p. 181-198.

[67] Hakamies-Blomqvist, L., T. Raitanen, and D. O'Neill, Driver ageing does not cause higher accident rates per km. Transportation Research Part F, 2002: p. 271-274.

[68] Langford, J., et al., Determining older driver crash responsibility from police and insurance data. Traffic Injury Prevention, 2006. 7(4): p. 343-351.

[69] Palumbo, A.J., et al., Driver licensing, motor-vehicle crashes, and moving violations among older adults. Journal of Safety Research, 2019. 71: p. 87-93.

[70] Koppel, S., et al., Older drivers, crashes and injuries. Traffic Injury Prevention, 2011. 12(5): p. 459-467.

[71] Daigneault, G., P. Joly, and J.Y. Frigon, Previous convictions or accidents and the risk of subsequent accidents of older drivers. Accident Analysis and Prevention, 2002. 34: p. 257-261.

[72] Ball, K.K., et al., Can high-risk older drivers be identified through performance-based measures in a Department of Motor Vehicles setting? Journal of the American Geriatrics Society, 2006. 54: p. 77-84.

[73] Clay, O.J., et al., Cumulative meta-analysis of the relationship between useful field of view and driving performance in older adults: Current and future implications. Optometry and Vision Science, 2005. 82(8): p. 724-731.

[74] Owsley, C., et al., Visual processing impairment and risk of motor vehicle crash among older adults. Journal of the American Medical Association, 1998. 279: p. 1083-1088.

[75] May, D., U.S.L. Nayak, and B. Isaacs, The life space diary: A measure of mobility in old people at home. International Rehabilitation Medicine, 1985. 7: p. 182-186.

[76] Parker, M., P.S. Baker, and R.M. Allman, A life-space approach to functional assessment of mobility in the elderly. Journal of Gerontological Social Work, 2001. 35(4): p. 35-55.

[77] Baker, P.S., E.V. Bodner, and R.M. Allman, Measuring life-space mobility in community-dwelling older adults. Journal of the American Geriatrics Society, 2003. 51(11): p. 1610-1614.

[78] Shoval, N., et al., The use of advanced tracking technologies for the analysis of mobility in Alzheimer's disease and related cognitive diseases. BMC Geriatrics, 2008. 26(8): p. 7.

[79] Barberger-Gateau, P. and C. Fabriguole, Disability and cognitive impairment in the elderly. Disability and Rehabilitation, 1997. 19(5): p. 175-193.

[80] Lochner, J.L., et al., Social isolation, support, and capital and nutritional risk in a older sample: Ethnic and gender differences. Social Science and Medicine, 2005. 60: p. 747-761.

[81] Barnes, L.L., et al., Correlates of life space in a volunteer cohort of older adults. Experimental Aging Research, 2007. 33(1): p. 77-93.

[82] Rantakokko, M., et al., Changes in life-space mobility and quality of life among community-dwelling older people: A 2-year follow-up study. Quality of Life Research, 2016. 25(5): p. 1189-1197.

[83] Crowe, M., et al., Life-space and cognitive decline in a community-based sample of African American and Caucasian older adults. Journals of Gerontology. Series A, Biological Sciences and Medical Sciences, 2008. 63(11): p. 1241-1245.

[84] Poranen-Clark, T., et al., Executive function and life-space mobility in old age. Aging Clinical and Experimental Research, 2018. 30(2): p. 145-151.

Chapter 3

Metabolic Syndrome as the First Stage of Eldership; the Beginning of Real Aging

Alexander V. Panov, Marina A. Darenskaya, Sergey I. Dikalov and Sergey I. Kolesnikov

Abstract

The history of active worldwide scientific research on mechanisms of aging and the age-associated diseases counts more than five decades. Of these, among the numerous theories of aging, at least 50 years dominated the free radical theory of aging. Since mitochondria were found to be the major producers of free radicals, the research on aging became largely centered on mitochondria. At the end of 80s of the 20th century, physicians have established a new nosological entity named "Metabolic syndrome" comprising several simultaneously existing symptoms and risk factors, which increase with age to 47% in men and 64% for women. The diagnosis of metabolic syndrome (MetS) requires simultaneous presence of at least three out of five medical conditions: visceral obesity, hypertension, high blood sugar, insulin resistance, low serum high-density lipoprotein accompanied with high serum triglycerides. However, from the beginning of the definition of MetS there was, and still is, a rather lovely debate, which of the symptoms must be considered as the main one. In spite of the enormous number of publications on both mechanisms of aging and MetS, there was relatively small progress in understanding the fundamental processes in these closely related problems. On the contrary, the mitochondrial free radical theory was found to be wrong in its current paradigms. In this Chapter we will discuss recent discoveries and hypotheses which open new perspectives in both theoretical and practical approaches to the problems of aging and MetS. We will show how aging and development of MetS are closely related to each other and the normal ontogenesis of human beings. Why men and women have different rates of aging and mechanisms of transition to MetS. We state that MetS is not just a cluster of symptoms, but one of the last steps of individual ontogenesis, namely the first step of eldership when the aging rate may increase manifold.

Keywords: aging, eldership, energy metabolism, fatty acid oxidation, isoprostane lipid peroxidation, mitochondrial DNA, metabolic syndrome, obesity, ontogenesis, oxidative stress, perhydroxyl radical, reactive oxygen species, ROS, superoxide radical, type 2 diabetes

1. Introduction

Everybody wants to live a long and healthy life. However, the universal laws of the Irreversible Thermodynamics drive changes in our bodies from the moment of birth, when a human baby has maximum information in his genes and minimum entropy in his body, through a series of consecutive changes to the last stage, when a human body has much less information left in the remaining old genes and maximum entropy in his body, which finally fails and the person dies.

We intentionally started our Chapter by mentioning the genetically predetermined stages of development of the human organism because, as it happened, the concept of ontogeny was somehow lost during the decades of research on mechanisms of aging and metabolic syndrome. As we will see, this approach gives completely different perspectives on the problems from the point of view of normal postembryonic ontogenesis.

The problems of aging and life longevity are not just medical problems, but are complex of fundamental biological problems, which comprise evolution, ontogenesis, genetics, epigenetics, and interactions with the environment. For this reasons, researchers studied aging and longevity starting from simple organisms like yeast and worms, then more complex laboratory animals, and even species like crocodiles and birds. Humans are, probably, much less studied in this respect than, say, mice and rats. To this day there are dozens of aging theories, which reflect the complexity of the problem. We mention only few of the relatively recent theories of aging: The heterochromatin loss model [1, 2]; adult stem cell and mesenchymal progenitor theory [3]; hormonal regulation of longevity in mammals [4]; telomere hypothesis of aging [5, 6]; epigenetic theory [7], and finally, currently the most popular and experimentally developed the free radical hypothesis of aging [8–21]. All theories of aging and longevity are interrelated, but so far, there is no generalizing theory. Therefore, we will start our discussions on human aging mechanisms from the currently most important theory of aging: the mitochondrial free radical theory.

2. The mitochondrial free radical theory of aging (MFRTA)

Initially proposed by Harman [8], the "Free Radical Hypothesis of Aging" was later transformed to the "Mitochondrial Free Radical Theory of Aging" (MFRTA), because mitochondria were found to be the main source of free radicals [9–14, 19, 22]. Collectively, the free radicals derived from oxygen were named "reactive oxygen species" (ROS).

In order to understand the logic of the worldwide research on aging development, it would be useful to look back on the intellectual and scientific background existing 40–50 years ago. After discovery that mitochondria generate oxygen radicals [23, 24], there was an excitement in finding the "universal mechanism" of all diseases. Therefore, for a long-time research on biological effects of ROS was titled "oxidative stress", of which aging was only one of many damaging effects of ROS. For some time, it was not realized that organs and tissues age at different pace, and that environmental conditions, such as radiation, air contamination or industrial pollutants may contribute to the aging process.

Importantly, for a long time any clear-cut specific markers of systemic aging were not known, except mutations of mitochondrial DNA (mtDNA). There is a strong parallelism between production of ROS and mutations of mtDNA [13, 14, 25]. Until recently, this parallelism was explained by a belief that hundreds of "naked" circular mtDNA molecules lie in the mitochondrial matrix and thus mtDNA is an easy target for free radicals. The accumulation in cells of mtDNA damaged by ROS progressively inactivates the DNA templates necessary to repair damaged mitochondria. As a result, the accumulation of mtDNA mutations acts as the aging clock [25].

Understandably, mutations of mtDNA became one of the most important factors in explaining mechanisms of aging, age-associated diseases and practically most major human diseases [25–29]. Only recently it was discovered that mtDNA are protected by the proteinaceous "shield", nucleoids, and that there is no proof for the free radical direct effects on mtDNA [30–33].

Production of ROS occurs not only in organs and tissues, but also in blood cells where radicals evidently have functions different from those in parenchymal cells. The "respiratory burst" of phagocytic cells, when they come in contact with bacteria or immune complexes, is important source of superoxide radicals ($O_2^{\bullet-}$). Phagocytic cells include neutrophils, monocytes, macrophages and eosinophils known to produce large amounts of $O_2^{\bullet-}$ [34].

In some cells, particularly in hepatocytes, the major source of ROS may be of extramitochondrial origin [35]. In the liver, both $O_2^{\bullet-}$ and H_2O_2 are produced during metabolism of xenobiotics by the microsomal P-450-monoxygenases [36], and in the course of catabolism of purine nucleotides and nucleosides by xanthine oxidoreductase [37]. Liver peroxisomes also produce large amounts of hydrogen peroxide during catabolism of very long chain fatty acids and polyunsaturated fatty acids [38]. However, in the liver both mitochondria and peroxisomes possess high catalase activity, which neutralizes hydrogen peroxide [38, 39]. In addition to catalase and superoxide dismutase (isoforms 1 and 2) high activities, liver has high activities of glutathione S-transferase (GST) and glutathione peroxidase [40, 41], and Prohibitin-1 [42], which enhance the liver's antioxidant system. For this reason, liver is relatively protected from deleterious effects of ROS, has high regenerative capacity [43] and, therefore, the rate of aging of this organ is much slower, as compared with other organs [44, 45]. Kidneys also rarely create problems for elderly people because they work constantly at a relatively even pace. In the actively working organs production of ROS is minimal [21]. The fastest rates of aging occur in those organs, which have a wide range of workloads, such as skeletal muscles, brain and heart. These organs have very high capacities in respiratory activity and ATP production to satisfy the organ's energy demands at high workloads. These organs usually have increased ROS production at lower workloads or at rest [21].

Thus, aging is not an evenly distributed over the body process. In addition, mechanisms of aging are distinct in different organs and tissues, and the causing aging oxidants in various organs and tissues can also be different. In order to clarify the last statement and for the sake of the following discussion on the shortcuts of the current paradigm of the MFRTA, we give a brief description of the major biological and environmental radicals and biologically active molecules.

2.1 Superoxide radical ($O_2^{\bullet-}$) and hydrogen peroxide (H_2O_2)

Superoxide radical ($O_2^{\bullet-}$) and hydrogen peroxide (H_2O_2) are quantitatively the main species of ROS that are produced constantly by the mitochondrial respiratory chain [21, 22]. Superoxide radicals serve also as a source for other ROS: hydroperoxyl radical, peroxynitrite, lipid radicals. The proportion of H_2O_2, produced at the sites of the respiratory chain is small [21], but the superoxide in many tissues rapidly dismutate to hydrogen peroxide by very high activities of superoxide dismutases in the cytosol (Cu,Zn-SOD1) and mitochondrial matrix (Mn-SOD2) [22, 46]. At the beginning of the mitochondrial free radical theory, superoxide radical was regarded as very dangerous [34]. However, soon it was realized that after $O_2^{\bullet-}$ leaves the membrane's lipid phase, small and negatively charged superoxide anion instantly acquires the hydration shell and thus loses most of its chemical activity [47]. In addition, due to the high activities of SOD1 and SOD2, present at micromolar concentrations, the superoxide radical half-life is very short (milliseconds) [22]. For this reason attention was shifted to other radicals, which can be formed from the superoxide and hydrogen peroxide. Nevertheless, $O_2^{\bullet-}$ can directly damage enzymes, which contain 4Fe-4S clusters by knocking out one Fe^{2+} atom and turning the 4Fe-4S cluster to inactive 3Fe-4S. A typical enzyme is aconitase, which is sensitive to inhibition by superoxide.

2.2 Hydroxyl radical ($^{\bullet}OH$)

Hydrogen peroxide (H_2O_2), which by itself is a rather harmless chemical, in the presence of transition metal ions Fe^{2+} and Cu^{1+} produces highly aggressive hydroxyl radical ($^{\bullet}OH$) [34]. However, $^{\bullet}OH$ is so active that it instantly reacts with any molecule it encounters (except water). For this reason $^{\bullet}OH$ half-life is only 10^{-9} sec [48] and under normal conditions it is not as harmful as initially believed. This radical is dangerous when formed in very large quantities, such as after exposure to radiation, or high concentration of H_2O_2 and transition metal poisoning. The latter situation is often observed in the experiments *in vitro*, but hardly takes place *in vivo,* since transition metals in the cells are always chelated.

2.3 Nitric oxide ($^{\bullet}NO$) and peroxynitrite ($OONO^-$)

Tissues, such as blood vessels endothelium, neurons and others, which possess tissue-specific nitric oxide synthases (eNOS), produce a free radical nitric oxide ($^{\bullet}NO$), an important cellular signaling molecule involved in many physiological and pathological processes. Formation of one molecule of $^{\bullet}NO$ requires two molecules of O_2, and since the $^{\bullet}NO$ half-life *in vivo* is about 7 sec., for the maintenance of a steady-state concentration of $^{\bullet}NO$ at 1 μM, the consumption of oxygen is very high, about 120 nanomol O_2 per 1 gram of tissue per1 minute [49]. For this reason, the physiologically sufficient steady state levels of $^{\bullet}NO$ can be formed only in the oxygen rich cells, like vascular endothelium, or well vascularized organs like brain. $^{\bullet}NO$ is a powerful vasodilator. The biological effects of $^{\bullet}NO$ can be inhibited due to its fast reaction with superoxide radical yielding a rather toxic product peroxynitrite ($OONO^-$) [50]. Peroxynitrite is a strong oxidant and nitrating agent, it interacts with lipids, DNA, and proteins via direct oxidative reactions or via indirect, radical-mediated mechanisms. *In vivo*, peroxynitrite generation represents an important pathogenic mechanism in conditions such as stroke, myocardial infarction, chronic heart failure, diabetes, circulatory shock, chronic inflammatory diseases, cancer, and neurodegenerative disorders [49, 51]. Peroxynitrite plays an important role in pathologies and aging of some organs and tissues, such as blood vessels and neurons, but being a rather strong anion, it hardly contributes to the systemic mechanism of aging, which we will discuss a little later. Nitric oxide is hydrophobic, but chemically weak radical, and, thus, also can be excluded from the systemic aging mechanism, which occur in the lipid phase of the inner mitochondrial membrane.

At this point, we have not discussed the protonated form of superoxide radical ($O_2^{\bullet-}$), namely hydroperoxyl radical ($^{\bullet}HO_2$) because it will be done in conjunctions with the description of polyunsaturated fatty acids (PUFA) autoxidation, named "Isoprostane Pathway of Lipid Peroxidation" (IPLP), which we propose as the main mechanism of aging in people with Metabolic syndrome.

2.4 Environmental biologically active molecules and radicals

Unlike the above described ROS, which are formed in the body and relatively well-studied, the biological effects of sun radiation and air pollutants involving singlet oxygen and ozone are less known. However, they are the major causes of accelerated aging of skin and lung epithelium. For this reason, we provide a brief description of toxic effects of these ROS.

2.4.1 Singlet oxygen

Singlet oxygen is the common name for the two metastable states of molecular oxygen, but the singlet $O_2{}^1\Delta g$ is the most active in biological systems. It has no unpaired electrons and therefore is not a radical, but upon excitation, one of the O_2 electrons shifts to a higher and unstable orbit, which makes it chemically more active than regular triplet O_2. *In vivo* O_2 to $O_2{}^1\Delta g$ excitation occurs when the sunlight fells on human skin containing several biological pigments, such as porphyrins or flavins. This is the reason of early skin aging and skin damages in people with abnormal porphyrin metabolism. Formation of singlet O_2 by sunlight occurs also *in vivo* in both lens and retina of the mammalian eye, which causes cataract and loss of vision [52]. Thus, wearing dark glasses and a hat, even in not very bright weather, will protect eyes from cataracts early development and skin from early aging. Studies of plants suggested that in photosynthetic systems one of the functions of polyenes and carotenoids is to protect plants from damages caused by singlet oxygen. Therefore, a carrot salad dressed with vegetable oil may have protective effect against complications caused by bright sunlight.

2.4.2 Ozone (O_3)

Ozone (O_3) is an allotrope of oxygen and is much less stable than normal O_2. It forms under the influence of ultraviolet light and during atmospheric electrical discharges (lightning). Even at low concentrations ozone causes damages to respiratory tracts of experimental animals and organic materials, such as latex and various types of plastic. The ozone's half-life depends on temperature, humidity and air circulation. In a closed room with running fan, ozone's half-life is about 24 hours [53]. That is, in a laboratory room, an instrument, like spectrophotometer or spectrophluorometer without special device for burning ozone (for example, instruments from Perkin Elmer), after several hours of work may create a concentration of ozone high enough to cause a headache and errors in experimental results due to accumulation of peroxides in water solutions.

2.4.3 Nitrogen dioxide ($^\bullet NO_2$)

For the human's health it is important that in industrial areas with chemical factories and coal power stations the air may be polluted with nitrogen dioxide that may damage skin and respiratory organs. $^\bullet NO_2$ induces oxidation, as well as cell's membrane proteins nitration. Nitrated biological products, for example, tyrosine-containing proteins and nitrolipids are often found in the body. It is likely, that $^\bullet NO_2$ has been involved in the formation of these products [54].

2.4.4 Peroxynitrates

Nitrogen dioxide quickly reacts with other radicals. This is one of nitrotyrosines formation important mechanisms. During reaction $^\bullet NO_2 + O_2^{\bullet-} \rightarrow O_2NOO^\bullet$ very rapidly forms peroxynitrate: It contributes to skin and lung damage mechanisms during their contact with air polluted with nitrogen dioxide [54].

3. Crisis of the mitochondrial free radical theory of aging (MFRTA)

From the described above different free radicals and environmental pollutants, we see that all of them have the potential ability to cause damages to cellular and mitochondrial functions, although by different mechanisms. Some of the biologically active molecules and radicals show clear tissue and organ specificities. For example, singlet oxygen damages predominantly skin and eyes; ozone and nitrogen dioxide - lung epithelium, nitric oxide and peroxynitrite - vascular endothelium and neuronal cells. However, none of the above ROS is directly related, with the exception of the superoxide radical, to the inevitable aging mechanism [55].

After decades of research a vast amount of accumulated knowledge revealed serious inconsistencies between the data obtained and the MFRTA, which call into question the correctness of the free radical theory in its current paradigms. We refer the reader to excellent reviews on this topic [16, 18, 56–58]. Taking into consideration the controversies regarding various species, in this Chapter we will focus only on those inconsistencies that directly relate to the topic of humans and mammalians aging mechanism. Animals are often used for modeling of aging mechanisms [59–62]. We shall discuss the following most important for MFRTA facts, which undermine this theory.

3.1 MtDNA are protected from the direct effects of reactive oxygen species

Recently, it has been established that neither of the above listed ROS and biologically active molecules are capable to cause directly mutations of mtDNA, which was and still is for many researchers the main hallmark of the aging process and it is considered as the main pathogenic mechanism of many diseases [30–33]. From the beginning of free radical theory of aging, mutations of mtDNA were the only reliable markers of oxidative stress. As a matter of fact, the MFRTA itself arose on the basis that changes in the production of ROS were always accompanied by parallel changes in the number of mtDNA mutations [13, 14, 25]. Recently, however, it was concluded that there was no reliable evidence for the direct involvement of ROS in mtDNA mutations [31, 57]. There are two main reasons for this conclusion. First, the commonly studied radicals are not active enough to cause mutations [55]. Secondly, mtDNA are encased into a protein coating of nucleoid, which prevents direct contact of mtDNA and radicals [31].

3.2 Antioxidant supplementation interventions do not increase longevity

Antioxidant supplementation interventions do not increase longevity, as would be predicted by the MFRTA. This Antioxidant Paradox is considered as the strongest evidence against the MFRTA; it comes from studies that manipulate antioxidant levels. Many studies have shown that administration of low-molecular weight antioxidants failed to extend longevity [reviewed in 16, 56, 57, 63]. Barja (2014) suggested that the lack of antioxidants to exert effects on longevity could be explained by the spatial separation: a free radical, which causes aging, acts in the lipid phase of membranes, while antioxidants exerts their effects mostly in the water phase of cells [16]. Barja (2014) also summarized the numerous studies of life longevities on various species: "Only two parameters currently correlate with species longevity in the right sense: the mitochondrial rate of reactive oxygen species (mitoROS) production and the degree of fatty acid unsaturation of tissue membranes" [16]. As we will see, these are very correct suggestions.

3.3 The rate of $O_2^{\bullet-}$ production controls lifespan independently of SOD

Muller (2000) has stressed that SOD activity interspecies variation is not correlated with the maximal life span (MLSP) in mammals and the activity of other antioxidant enzymes negatively correlates with MLSP. However, there is a strong negative correlation between longevity and the $O_2^{\bullet-}$ and H_2O_2 production rates by isolated mitochondria from diverse mammalian species. The longevity depends not on the amount of superoxide in a cell, but on the rate of its production [18]. To explain this unexpected observation, Muller suggested that a significant fraction (between 10% and 50%) of $O_2^{\bullet-}$ is not produced as aqueous $O_2^{\bullet-}$ but instead is produced as lipid-phase $HO_2^{\bullet}$ in the inner mitochondrial membrane. In other words, Muller has proposed that it is not the $O_2^{\bullet-}$ in the water phase, but its protonated form - hydroperoxyl radical ($HO_2^{\bullet}$) in the membrane lipid phase exerts damaging effects on longevity, where the radical cannot be affected by a superoxide dismutase. Muller suggested that hydroperoxyl radical may initiate lipid peroxidation and the formation of peroxynitrous acid [18]. Unfortunately, the proposal that the hydroperoxyl radical is the aging main cause remained unnoticed for the next two decades, as well as the earlier similar attempts of other researchers before Muller [48, 63].

4. Hydroperoxyl radical $HO_2^{\bullet}$ as the systemic aging cause

Here we present in brief our current views on the mechanisms of the hydroperoxyl radical formation and its damaging effects, which we consider as the systemic aging main mechanism. The details of the mechanism are presented in recent publications [55, 64–67].

5. Properties of the hydroperoxyl radical or perhydroxyl radical ($^{\bullet}HO_2$)

Lipid phase of the mitochondrial membrane has 4–5 fold higher concentration of oxygen than the cells' water in the cytosol. When O_2 acquires an electron from the respiratory chain and becomes $O_2^{\bullet-}$, it must quickly leave the lipid phase of the membrane. However, before $O_2^{\bullet-}$ riches the bulk of the matrix or cytosol, it crosses the thing layer of the structured water near the charged surfaces of the membrane. The inner leaflet of the inner mitochondrial membrane contains approximately 80–90% of total cardiolipin (CL), which, together with phosphatidylethanolamine (PEA), accommodate respiratory complexes and ATP-synthase into the mitochondrial cristae sharp curves [67]. Since CL bears strong negative charge, at some arears of the inner membrane aggregates of CL form areas with strong negative charge, called antennae, which attract protons [reviewed in 66, 68]. For this reason, the thin layer of structured water near the charged surfaces of the inner mitochondrial membrane has up to three units more acid pH than the bulk of a compartment. This is a very important issue, because 1000 times higher concentration of H^+ increases the probability of the hydroperoxyl radical formation in the $O_2^{\bullet-} + H^+ \leftrightarrow {}^{\bullet}HO_2$ reversible reaction (pK_α of the reaction is 4.8) [68]. Highly hydrophobic $^{\bullet}HO_2$ returns back into the membrane's lipid phase. The described mechanism explains why the aging process depends only on the rate of superoxide formation, but not on the concentration of $O_2^{\bullet-}$ and the activities of SODs. Hydroperoxyl radical is a much stronger oxidizing agent than superoxide radical, and has a specific propensity to abstract H atoms from α-tocopherol and, particularly, from the polyunsaturated fatty acids, such as arachidonic acid (C20:4 n6) and docosahexaenoic acid (C22:6 n3) [69].

For unknown reason, the perhydroxyl radical for a long time was almost completely excluded from the oxidative stress literature [61, 70]. Mitchell (2000) proposed perhydroxyl radical damaging mechanism through formation of peroxynitrite radical in the membrane [18]. This possible situation has been discussed by Gebicki and Bielski [69]. These authors indicated that although both $^{\bullet}NO$ and $^{\bullet}HO_2$ are hydrophobic radicals, the radicals are spatially separated since $^{\bullet}NO$ is normally present in the blood vessel endothelium, and thus the mitochondrial hydroperoxyl radicals have little chance to meet nitric oxide, and even if this might happen, the negatively charged $ONOO^-$ hardly could be a systemic damaging factor because it is immediately excluded from the membrane's lipid phase [69]. Bielski et al. (1983) studied reactions of $^{\bullet}HO_2$ with linoleic (C18:2), linolenic (C18:3) and arachidonic acids (C20:4) in water/ethanol solutions [68]. The obtained kinetic parameters of the reactions indicate that $^{\bullet}HO_2$ reacts with the double allyl hydrogens of polyunsaturated fatty acids, and the more double bonds was present in a PUFA, the more active was the reaction. The abstraction of H atoms by $^{\bullet}HO_2$ was exothermic, which indicates that it is irreversible and highly probable, when $^{\bullet}HO_2$ encounters a PUFA. Since the reactions were performed in the water/ethanol solution, H_2O_2 formed cleaved heterolytically ($2H_2O_2 \rightarrow H_2O + O_2$), and the final products of the fatty acids with $^{\bullet}HO_2$ reactions were stable hydroperoxides without much variation in their structure [68].

6. The isoprostane pathway of lipid peroxidation (IPLP)

When $^{\bullet}HO_2$ reacts inside the lipid phase of the membrane with a PUFA, which is still part of a phospholipid, the products are a racemic mixture of a very large number of various stereo- and positional isomers [71]. Many of these products are similar to enzymatically produced prostaglandins, and were named Isoprostanes (IsoPs). For this reason, this type of PUFA autoxidation was named the Isoprostane Pathway of Lipid Peroxidation (IPLP) [71–73]. IsoPs possess potent biological activity and thus may convey abnormal cellular signaling and inflammation [71, 74]. Furthermore, many products of IPLP are very toxic, such as γ-ketoaldehydes. They form adducts with primary amines of the lysine-containing proteins and phosphatidylethanolamine (PEA). The most active among γ-ketoaldehydes are isolevuglandins (IsoLG) produced from arachidonic acid can be only detected as adducts with proteins or ethanolamine of PEA [74]. In addition to arachidonic acid the most common PUFA among phospholipids, other PUFA such as eicosapentaenoic acid (20:5 n3) and docosahexaenoic acid (22:6 n3), have been found as substrates for the IPLP [75]. Because docosahexaenoic acid (DHA) is present in a larger quantity in neurons, the products of IPLP were correspondingly named neuroprostanes and neuroketals. From arachidonic acid, which has four double bonds, the racemic mixture may contain up to eight hundreds of different products, whereas the products number from the containing 6 double bonds docosahexaenoic acid may be more than one thousand [71–73].

IsoPs and the cyclooxygenase derived prostaglandins (PGs) have a number of distinctions in their origin and properties, which have been discussed in a number of publications [65, 71, 76, 77]. Here we briefly list the most important distinctions: 1) The side chains of normal PGs are almost always oriented *trans* to the prostane ring whereas the products of IPLP have mostly the side chains with *cis* orientation [71, 76]; 2) The IsoPs are formed *in situ* from PUFA, which are esterified to phospholipids, while PGs are generated exclusively from the free AA and DHA [77]. 3) The products of IPLP are the racemic mixture of molecules with a very large number of possible stereo- and positional isomers, whereas the products of the enzymatically produced prostaglandins have mainly one optical isomer [71, 76].

Figure 1A very schematically presents the pathways of arachidonic acid oxidation, and **Figure 1B** illustrates the suggested mechanism of AA oxidation by $^{\bullet}HO_2$ [65]. The key event after abstraction of the first H atom is that H_2O_2 formed under hydrophobic condition undergoes homolytic cleavage with formation of two molecules of the hydroxyl radicals $H_2O_2 \rightarrow 2\ ^{\bullet}OH$, which instantly subtract another two H atoms from the same PUFA with formation of two molecules of H_2O. The remaining molecule of the AA has completely disarranged double bonds, becomes extremely unstable and quickly attaches randomly two O_2 molecules, and undergoes intramolecular transitions with formation of one out of many possible positional and stereoisomers. Thus $^{\bullet}HO_2$ converts into 2 H_2O and AA loses two out of 4 double bonds, and becomes one of hundreds isoprostanes. The differences between IPLP and the "classical" lipid peroxidation have been discussed in [65, 79].

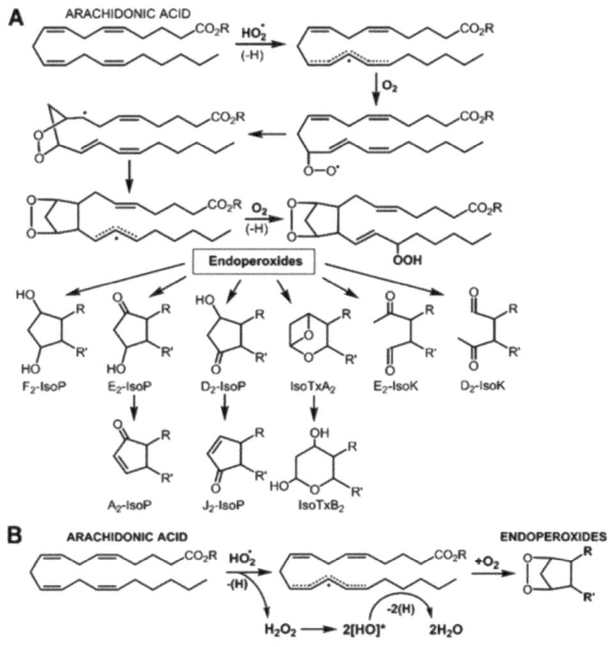

Figure 1.
Autoxidation of arachidonic acid with transformation of the molecule into various ring structures. (A) this part of the figure was adapted from the article [78] and shows different intermediary metabolites during autoxidation of arachidonic acid (AA). $HO_2^{\bullet}$ is the only candidate for initiation of the isoprostane autoxidation of PUFA [65]. (B) the suggested sequence of transformations of $HO_2^{\bullet}$ and AA in the course of isoprostane lipid peroxidation (IPLP) [65]. After abstraction of the first H atom from a molecule of AA, $HO_2^{\bullet}$ turns into H_2O_2, which in the hydrophobic milieu undergoes homolytic cleavage into two molecules of $^{\bullet}OH$ radicals, which instantly subtract the next two H atoms from the AA with formation of two molecules of H_2O and the remains of the AA has completely disarranged double bonds. A very fast abstraction of three H atoms from any of the four double bonds leads to the fact that the residue of the AA becomes extremely unstable and quickly attaches two O_2 molecules in a random way and undergoes intramolecular transitions with formation of one out of many possible positional and stereoisomers. The more PUFA has double bonds, the more possible isomers for the end product of the reaction. Abbreviations: F_2-IsoP, E_2-IsoP, D_2-IsoP – Isoprostanes with, correspondingly, prostane rings F_2, E_2, D_2 or A_2 and J_2; $IsoTxA_2$ and $IsoTxB_2$ – Isothromboxanes with rings A_2 и B_2, correspondingly, which were formed from prostaglandins H_2 (PGH_2); E_2-IsoK и D_2-IsoK – Isoketals with rings E_2 и D_2.

7. IPLP as the mechanism of aging

It has been demonstrated by researchers from the Vanderbilt University that IsoPs are the most early and reliable markers of lipid peroxidation *in vivo*, and recent studies provided valuable information about participation of IPLP in pathogenesis of numerous human diseases [80–82]. According to our model of IPLP initiation by $HO_2^•$, the hydroperoxyl radical upon encounter with a PUFA produces one of many variants of isoPG, γ-ketoaldehyde or isolevuglandins. When reacting with fatty acids with two unsaturated bonds, such as linoleic acids of cardiolipin, $HO_2^•$ produces corresponding hydroperoxides.

The different toxic products of the IPLP evidently cause numerous and different lesions to mitochondria gradually causing wear and tear of mitochondrial and cellular functions. We distinguish two types of direct lesions to mitochondria: one dysfunctions type is caused by oxidation of CL and PEA, which result in structural changes of respirosomes and ATP-synthase complexes. The second dysfunctions type is caused by direct damages by toxic products, like isolevuglandins, which directly form adducts with PEA and lysine of proteins. This type of damages may explain mtDNA replication damages [33, 34, 83]. Anderson et al. [83] have shown that mtDNA replicase *exo* domain, Pol gamma, is far more sensitive to oxidation than *pol* domain. The authors suggested that under oxidative conditions, exonuclease activity therefore declines more rapidly than polymerase. The oxidized Pol gamma becomes editing-deficient, displaying a 20-fold elevated mutations than the unoxidized enzyme [83]. PEA may be damaged by both pathways: via PUFA at C2 autoxidation, and via formation of adducts of ethanolamine with IsoLG produced upon activation if IPLP by $HO_2^•$. Of note, most of the ROS have very short lifetime (seconds) but IsoLG produce rather stable adducts (lifetime days), which can accumulate with age and, therefore, contribute to the development of age-associated conditions.

8. The importance of fatty acids oxidation for increased rate of ROS production

Mammalian tissues mitochondria generate superoxide and hydrogen peroxide (ROS) from 11 different sites depending on substrates used and the redox state of the electron transport chain [21]. All mitochondrial ROS production sites have distinct properties [21, 84]. They can be divided into two groups: six sites operate at the redox potential of the NADH/NAD^+ isopotential pool, about −280 mV, and five sites operate at the redox potential of the ubiquinol/ubiquinone (QH_2/Q) isopotential pool, about +20 mV [21, 84].

Much of the published literature on contribution of separate respiratory complexes in generation of ROS have potential problems for several reasons: first, the authors often used inhibitors of the respiratory chain, which is far from situation *in situ*, secondly, most authors used a single substrate, whereas *in situ* mitochondria metabolize several substrates simultaneously [85–88]. Most importantly and, with few exceptions, authors never used fatty acids as substrates for mitochondrial respiration. Brandt and colleagues provided evidence that the highest rates of ROS production ($O_2^{•-}$ + H_2O_2) are observed during β-oxidation of fatty acids [21, 84, 89]. During β-oxidation of fatty acids the membrane's pool of CoQ becomes fully reduced to $CoQH_2$ and this may reverse the transport of reducing equivalents at the level of succinate dehydrogenase (SDH), also known as Complex II, and thus activate the reverse electron transport and involve the sites of respiratory Complexes I and III, and SDH (Complex II) in production of ROS [21, 89].

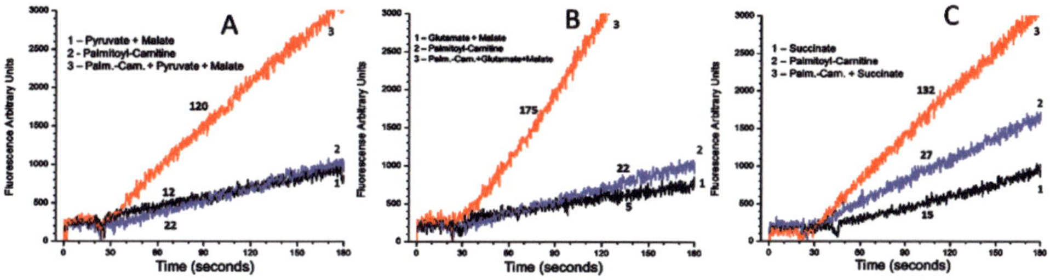

Figure 2.
Production of superoxide radicals by rat heart mitochondria oxidizing palmitoyl-carnitine. Designations: 1. Supporting substrate only; 2. Palmitoyl-carnitine only, and 3. Palmitoyl-carnitine + supporting substrate. Substrates: ***Figure 2A*** *- pyruvate 2.5 mM + malate 2 mM,* ***Figure 2B*** *- glutamate 5 mM + malate 2 mM, and* ***Figure 2C****. – Succinate 5 mM. Experimental conditions are described in [88]. The incubation medium contained: Amplex red 2 μM, horse radish peroxidase 2 units, substrates as indicated above, volume 1 ml. The reaction was initiated by addition of 50 μg of mitochondria. Initial rates were measured for 3 minutes. Numbers at the traces are the rates of H_2O_2 production in picomol H_2O_2/min/mg protein RHM. The rates were corrected for the time control rate with RHM incubated without added substrates. The figure was taken from [88].*

It has been recently shown that active oxidation of palmitoyl-carnitine by mitochondria in all metabolic states absolutely requires the simultaneous presence of any of the other mitochondrial metabolites such as: pyruvate, succinate, malate or glutamate, which were designated as "fatty acid oxidation supporting substrates" [87, 88]. In the presence of supporting substrates, fatty acids are actively oxidized not only by the isolated heart mitochondria [88], but also by the brain synaptic mitochondria [87], which breaks the old myth that the brain's energy metabolism is supported almost exclusively by glucose [reviewed in 87].

Most importantly, active oxidation of fatty acids in the presence of supporting substrates results in a manifold increase in ROS production in resting mitochondria (**Figure 2**). Earlier, we have proposed that oxidative damages and thus accelerated aging, are more common for organs, which have a wide range of physiological activities, such as heart, skeletal muscles and brain [65, 88]. When these organs are at low workloads or at rest, the very efficient oxidation of fatty acids may redirect excessive electrons to generation of ROS.

9. OK, MRFTA is valid, but what is aging?

In the sections above, we presented evidence that in spite of complications of the MFRTA based on old paradigms, the latest discoveries clearly support the essence of this theory, and the introduction of the perhydroxyl radical as a new mediator of oxidative stress resolve most of the contradictions. However, MFRTA still requires further consideration and we have to find answers to simple questions: what is aging and when the aging begins?

From the beginning, researchers working on MFRTA held the point of view that aging is a pathological process caused by oxidative stress that affects our health, and over time, we succumb to a myriad of age-related pathologies and eventually die [12, 58]. But is aging simply the process of errors accumulation? The Dictionary of Science and Technology designates aging as "the process of growing older or changing over time" [90]. In other words, a person after birth goes through a series of genetically controlled transitions, which are called postembryonic ontogenesis [91]. From the point of view of a human ontogeny, we can roughly divide a person's individual life into five periods: infancy, childhood, adolescence, reproductive period and post-reproductive, or aging period. For several reasons, we hardly expect that during infancy, childhood and adolescence "a myriad of age-related pathologies" might be accumulated [58]. We will consider the last two periods: "reproductive", which comprises the ages from 20 to 50, and the "aging period", which begins after the age of 50 [92].

Among recent definitions of aging there were few in more general terms: "Aging is characterized by a gradual decline in various health parameters across multiple biochemical, physiological and behavioral systems" [93]. Correspondingly, some researchers started looking for a subset of aging individuals with lack of resilience within these general physiological systems, a condition termed frailty. Frailty has been defined in broad terms as an age-associated syndrome characterized by increased vulnerability to external influences, a diminished capacity to respond correctly to stressors and as an overall loss of fitness. In general, frail individuals are at a greater risk of falls, dependency, disability, institutionalization, hospitalization and mortality [94]. Frailty can be measured in relation to the accumulation of deficits using a frailty index. A frailty index can be developed from most aging databases [95, 96].

In another parallel world of Science, a large group of researchers study the metabolic syndrome, a nosological entity established at the end of 80s of the last century. The metabolic syndrome (MetS) was defined as a condition of simultaneous existence of several risk factors, including obesity, insulin resistance, atherogenic dyslipidemia and hypertension, which are interrelated, age-dependent, and share underlying mediators and metabolic pathways [97]. Undoubtedly, both concepts of frailty and metabolic syndrome are important from a medical perspective, but apparently did little for understanding the mechanisms of aging. Due to intensive research on both concepts, however, there has been made a great discovery: the rates of aging and energy metabolism are sex-specific. In our opinion, these discoveries are crucial for understanding the mechanisms of aging as the process of transition of an individual from the reproduction period to the last stage of ontogeny – aging.

10. Sex-specific differences in the rates of aging and longevity

Most animals and plants are sexual, in spite of the reproductive advantages experienced by asexual variants. Evidently there where selective forces that gave an advantage to sexuality and genetic recombination at either the population or individual level. The effect of sex and recombination increases the efficiency of natural selection, which is a major factor favoring evolution [98, 99]. It has been experimentally shown that sex increases the rate of adaptation to a new harsh environment, but has no measurable effect on fitness in a new benign environment where there is little selection [100]. Nonetheless, we are still far from a definitive answer to the question of why sexual reproduction is so common [99]. Recently, the hypothesis has been put forward that the internal production of ROS 2 billion years ago started the eukaryotic sex (re)evolution [101]. It has also been stressed that earlier theoretical works on sexual reproduction ignored important complexities that face natural populations, such as genetic drift and the spatial structure of populations [102].

The data accumulated show that in many species, including humans, females have slower rate of aging and longer life span than males [99, 103–105]. We suggest that this observation has important general biological goals for a female: bearing and raising a new generation despite any external difficulties and metabolic restrictions. These goals demand that females have to be efficient enough, but not superefficient from the metabolic (thermodynamic) point of view, resilient to harsh environmental conditions, and, in accord with the MFRTA, have lower rate of oxidative stress. Numerous studies of various species showed that in general females have slower production of ROS than males [99]. As always, there are some exclusions from the general rule, but again they hold the same conclusion: the longer living gender produces less ROS [106].

In the next sections we will discuss possible mechanisms underlying the slower aging and slower rates of ROS production in the longer living females.

11. Sex-specific differences in the rates of fat utilization for the sake of energy metabolism

Laboratory animals are indispensable part of biomedical research and widely used for modeling physiological and pathological situations in humans [107]. For ethical and technical restrictions, it is impossible to study many biomedical problems on humans, whereas animal research provides a degree of experimental control and precision not usually feasible in studies using human subjects [108]. Meanwhile, the animals used in most experiments were males, because researchers usually avoid using females for the reason of their reproductive cycles and hormone fluctuations that may affect the results of their studies [109]. For these reasons research on sex differences has begun relatively recently, but today the related literature is enormous. Human studies on metabolic differences between men and women were stimulated largely due to the progress of the sport medicine. Here, we will discuss only those works, which have direct relation to our subject under discussion: what sex metabolic differences underlie the fact that females live longer than males in many species, including humans [108].

Evidently, the sex differences in the body structure and metabolism depend on the stage of a person's ontogeny. Vijay et al. (2015) studied sexual differences in the expression of mitochondria-related genes in rat heart at different ages that correspond to different stages of the rat's reproductive capacities [110]. The authors studied the whole genome expression profiling in the hearts of young (8-week), adult (21-week), and old (78-week) male and female Fischer 344 rats, and the expression of 670 unique genes related to various mitochondrial functions was analyzed. A significant ($p < 0.05$) sexual dimorphism in expression was observed in young animals for 46, adult for 114 and old rats for 41 genes, respectively [110]. Importantly, in young and adult hearts, sexual dimorphism was not noted in genes encoding oxidative phosphorylation. Adult males showed higher expression of genes associated with the pyruvate dehydrogenase complex as compared to females. In old rats a majority of genes involved in oxidative phosphorylation had higher expression in females. This clearly shows that sexual dimorphism largely depends on the stage of ontogeny. Other studies demonstrated better preservation of myocardial mass and a greater cardiac contractility in women than men during aging [111]. The better heart health in aged women might be the result of either genetically predetermined factors or less oxidative damages and slower aging as compared to men.

It is a well-known observation that women generally have a higher amount of body fat than men. Distribution of fat is also different: women store more fat in the gluteal-femoral region, whereas men have more body fat in the abdominal (visceral) region [112, 113]. Importantly, that visceral fat accumulation is accompanied with multiple endocrine perturbations, including elevated cortisol and androgens in women, as well as low growth hormone and, in men, testosterone secretion. The consequences of the hormones effects will be more expressed in visceral than subcutaneous adipose tissues, because omental fat has higher cellularity, innervation and blood flow. Furthermore, the density of cortisol and androgen receptors seems to be higher in visceral fat than in other regions of adipose tissue [114]. In addition, there are epidemiological and metabolic associations between centralized (visceral) fat accumulation and disease [114]. This is an important fact because visceral obesity is a common symptom for men and women with metabolic syndrome.

Physiological experiments with oral administration of triglycerides, labeled with a small amount of oleic acid, revealed the following regional differences in the order of lipid uptake: omental = retroperitoneal > subcutaneous abdominal > subcutaneous femoral adipose tissues in men, with a similar rank order for half-life of the triglyceride, indicating also a turn-over of triglycerides in that order. Testosterone amplifies these differences in men. In premenopausal women, the visceral fat accumulation is smaller than in men, and subcutaneous abdominal has a higher turnover than femoral adipose tissue [114]. Among regional gender differences of fat metabolism, there is an interesting evidence that *in vivo*, catecholamine mediated leg free fatty acid release is lower in women than in men, whereas free fatty acid release from the upper body depots is comparable [112].

These experiments *in vivo* indicate that sex variations in fat metabolism are controlled by sex-specific hormones. This presumes that in the post-reproductive stage of ontogenesis, the sexual dimorphism in fat metabolism should be weaker or absent. Results of studies *in vitro* also indicate that this difference is diminished at the menopause, and may be restored by estrogen therapy. This suggest that the functional effects of estrogens in women are similar to those of testosterone in men. As we will show in the next section, the effects of both hormones are targeted on substrate oxidations by mitochondria, and, thus, on the rates of ROS production. However, the mechanism of estrogen on fat metabolism might be indirect because human adipose tissue does not possess specific estrogen and progesterone receptors [114].

As regards protein metabolism, no gender differences in the basal level net muscle protein balance have been found [115]. In general, testosterone increases muscle protein synthesis and net muscle protein balance, resulting in increased muscle mass. At young age, boys and girls have similar amounts of testosterone. At puberty testosterone levels increase much more dramatically in males, as does muscle mass. Furthermore, although no evidence exists in humans, the in-vitro and rat data suggest that ovarian hormones inhibit muscle protein synthesis [115].

12. Sex differences in substrate utilization during physical activities

The indirect effect of the sex hormones on fat metabolism is supported by the data on sexual dimorphism in utilization of fatty acids during physical activities, which demonstrate that the proportion of energy derived from fat during exercise is higher in women than in men [112, 116]. Carter et al. (2001) investigated the effect of endurance training on whole body substrate, glucose, and glycerol utilization during 90 min of exercise in males and females [116]. First, during submaximal physical loads females show a lower respiratory exchange ratio (RER) than males, which indicates on a proportionately lower carbohydrate and higher fat oxidation [116, 117]. In comparison with females, exercising males had a greater increase in leucine oxidation but not lysine levels, which indicated that during intensive physical activity males increase their need for amino acids to fuel energy needs. Under the same conditions, females responded by increased mobilization of fat, thereby requiring less alternative fuels such as carbohydrate and amino acids [116–118]. The overall conclusion of these experiments was that females oxidize a greater proportion of fat and less carbohydrates and amino acids as compared with males. Thus physiologists support our finding that fatty acids oxidation requires simultaneous presence of other mitochondrial metabolites derived from carbohydrates or proteins [88]. Because women have lesser consumption of supporting substrates, the rate of fatty acids oxidation should be also diminished. This might explain why, in general, women demonstrate lower levels of physical performance during endurance sports and produce less ROS [119–121].

Knowing the fact that mitochondria oxidize fatty acids only in the presence of supporting substrates [87, 88], the data presented above suggest that females require less or different supporting substrates for effective oxidation of fatty acids. We can, therefore, predict that the isolated skeletal muscle or heart mitochondria from females must be different from males in terms of the type and requirement of supporting substrates, and also produce ROS at a slower rate. Unfortunately, until now we have been the only ones who have studied the oxidation of fatty acids in the presence of various supporting substrates, but we used male rats only in our experiments [87, 88]. **Figure 3** illustrates that the rates of ROS production strongly depend on the type of supporting substrates, namely pyruvate, glutamate and succinate, and their various mixtures [55, 87, 88]. Thus the *in vitro* experiments with the isolated mitochondria from different organs require further investigation in order to elucidate molecular mechanisms of the sex diversity at the mitochondrial level. Since males showed higher expression of genes associated with the pyruvate dehydrogenase complex, as compared to females [111], and consume more carbohydrates and amino acids during endurance training [116–118] we can suggest that women's higher longevity and slower rate of aging is associated with the less efficient oxidation of fatty acids and thus slower rates of oxidative stress. However, this conclusion evidently regards only women at the reproductive stage, when, according to Ventura-Clapier et al. (2020), women are "protected" [122]. These authors also stated that "apart from comparisons between males and females, there is a crucial need for studying the female physiology and woman pathology. In particular the biological step that constitutes menopause in women appears to be the border between "female protection" and "female susceptibility" to cardiovascular diseases, which needs to be deciphered further".

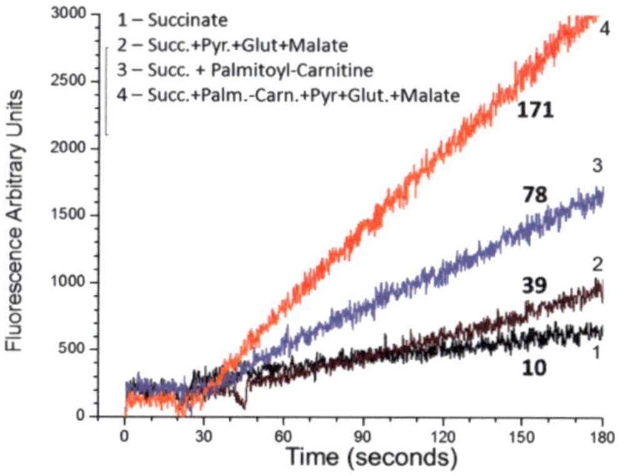

Figure 3.
Effect of substrate mixtures on production of ROS by isolated rat heart mitochondria oxidizing palmitoyl-carnitine. The incubation medium contained: Amplex red 2 μM, horse radish peroxidase 2 units, volume 1 ml. The reaction was initiated by addition of 50 μg of mitochondria. Initial rates were measured for 3 minutes. Substrates: 1. Succinate 5 mM; 2. Succinate + pyruvate 2.5 mM + glutamate 5 mM + malate 2 mM; 3. Palmitoyl-carnitine 50 μM + succinate; 4. Palmitoyl-carnitine + succinate + pyruvate + glutamate + malate. Numbers at the traces are the rates of H_2O_2 production in picomol H_2O_2/min/mg protein RHM. The rates were corrected for the time control rate with RHM incubated without added substrates. The figure was taken from [55].

13. Metabolic syndrome (MetS) as the post-reproductive stage of ontogenesis

Long time ago physicians noticed that many patients have common features of external appearances and biochemical indices of abnormal metabolism, which included insulin resistance, obesity, atherogenic dyslipidemia and hypertension. By the end of 80s of the 20th century the term "Metabolic syndrome" has been accepted and its own diagnostic code: 277.7 has been assigned by the International Classification, 9th Division, Clinical Modification (ICD-9-CM). However, the current definitions of the metabolic syndrome (MetS) give no clues to the essence of MetS and are mostly just listings of symptoms, for example: "The metabolic syndrome is a constellation of metabolic disorders including obesity, hypertension, and insulin resistance, components, which are risk factors for the development of diabetes, hypertension, cardiovascular, and renal disease" [123, 124]. This "clustering" or "constellation" of risk factors were considered to share underlying causes, mechanisms and features. The diagnosis of MetS is accepted only when at least three out of five symptoms are present in a patient [125, 126]. It was early recognized that people with isolated components, but who do not fit the definition of metabolic syndrome, are not at as high a risk for type 2 diabetes (T2D) or cardiovascular diseases (CVD). For example, people with isolated hypertension or isolated hyperlipidemia are at risk of CVD, or people with isolated obesity are at risk for T2D, but less so than people who meet multiple criteria of MetS [123].

It was expected that a comprehensive definition for the metabolic syndrome and its key features will facilitate research into its causes and lead to pharmacologic and lifestyle treatment approaches [127]. However, analysis of the tremendous amount of publications regarding MetS revealed that more than 30 years after defining MetS, there is still no deep understanding how and why MetS develops. Much of the literature can be roughly divided into supporters and opponents of considering insulin resistance as the primary symptom for the diagnosing MetS [123, 128–130]. These discrepancies were reflected in the criteria for diagnosing MetS provided by several Institutions, which were thoroughly reviewed in [123]. The discussions become heated by publications that ethnic and racial factors may greatly affect the criteria for diagnosis of MetS [127, 131].

14. The origin of MetS

The results of genetics studies on the potential hereditary predisposition to MetS were analyzed by Stančakova and Laakso [132]. They concluded that there is only a limited evidence for common genetic background explaining the clustering of the metabolic trait. Instead, the existing evidence suggests the importance of epigenetic mechanisms [132]. This conclusion supports our earlier suggestion [55, 66, 67] that the external appearances and metabolic features of MetS reflect the genetic properties of our distant ancestors. So far, however, aging and MetS have been commonly regarded as the result of accumulation of different kinds of damages caused by oxidative stress and/or improper life style [8–11, 133–135].

As we have stressed earlier, all human beings after birth undergo changes during postembryonic ontogenesis. One of the theories of aging suggests that with the advanced age, the loss of heterochromatin results in altered gene expression [1, 2]. The epigenetic alterations resulting from global heterochromatin loss may be at the root of the various molecular events associated with aging and may tie together the various models of aging [2]. However, the process of ontogenesis in humans suggests that each transition to a new stage switches conversion of a new portion of heterochromatin into euchromatin, and new genes begin to work, and then during transition to a the next stage, the "previous" portion of euchromatin does not turn back into heterochromatin, but becomes lost. Therefore, the so called "general loss" of the heterochromatin with advancing age simply reflects the advancement of individual ontogeny. Evidently, when men and women enter the post-reproductive stage of ontogenesis, they have lost much of the heterochromatin that was present in a newborn baby. The genes that govern the post-reproductive stage were not the subject for natural selection, and therefore they are the same, or almost the same, genes that our distant ancestors had. This can be proved by many qualities in our bodies that appear after the age of 55: bulky body structure, dark spots of myelin in the skin, hair distribution, etc. Evidently, after transition to the post-reproductive stage many metabolic features also become distinct from the previous stages. There is a lot of evidence that elderly people of the northern Europe and Siberia acquire external and metabolic features common to the people living in the Northern Polar Regions. Inhabitants of the North, for example Eskimos, Dolgans, Innuits, do not consume a lot of plant foods rich in carbohydrates. Their diet is based on meat, animal fat and fish.

Again, the clue to understanding the nature of MetS, we can find in the sex associated differences in the energy metabolism and the transition of men and women from reproductive to the post-reproductive stage of ontogenesis, which is commonly regarded as the stage of aging [92]. This usually occurs between the ages of 50 and 55, when women go through menopause. The sharp changes in appearance and metabolism are particularly evident in women during and after the menopause, which increases the risk of MetS by 60% [136]. It is important, that the occurrence of MetS in the post-menopause period does not depend on the body mass index (BMD) and physical activity [137], but may depend in women on the dynamics of estrogen decline with age [138]. Interestingly, studies on sex hormone replacement in animals have shown that males receiving testosterone showed MetS deterioration, while females with estrogen replacement showed improvement in their MetS symptoms such as decreased hypertension [139]. This agrees with the suggestion that the genetically predetermined transition to the post-reproductive stage during normal ontogenesis, which is accompanied by changes in the hormone status, is the major natural cause of MetS. Thus some features of MetS, namely insensitivity to insulin and gain of fat, particularly visceral obesity, simply reflect a new type of metabolism. From this point of view, T2D may result from the excessive consumption of unnecessary carbohydrates at the post-reproductive stage.

15. Sex differences in the transition from reproductive to post-reproductive stage

In one of the previous sections we provided evidence that women oxidize fatty acids, which are the predominant energy source at all ages, at a slower rate in comparison with men, and thus probably produce ROS at a slower rate [116–118]. Olivetty et all. [111] studied changes in mononucleated and binucleated myocytes with age in enzymatically dissociated cells. The age interval examined varied from 17 to 95 years. The authors have found that in the course of aging women's hearts preserved the ventricular myocardial mass, aggregate number of mononucleated and binucleated myocytes, average cell diameter and volume. In contrast, in the men's hearts the authors observed nearly 1 g/year loss of myocardium, and this phenomenon accounted for the loss of approximately 64 million cells. These detrimental events involved the whole male's heart. In the remaining cells, myocyte cell volume increased at a rate of 158 microns3/year in the left and 167 microns3/year in the right ventricle. And these changes in the men's hearts were linear from the age of 17 to 95, whereas in women the structural properties of the heart remained unchanged [111]. Thus, it seems that women enter the post-reproductive stage with relatively "young" heart, whereas in men the aged heart lost many cells and the remaining cells increased their volume, which is a disadvantage for the heart's energy metabolism.

16. Features of fatty acids metabolism that increase MetS symptoms and accelerate aging

Among mammalians the human females have a unique duration of post-reproductive longevity [140], which is probably to a large degree associated with the metabolic "protection" that caused slower rate of aging at the reproductive period [122]. There are several reasons to argue that both the accelerated rate of aging of men and the relatively slow aging of women, as well as other sex differences in metabolism and physical performance, are based on the sex differences in fatty acids metabolism. Regardless of age and gender, fats are the major source of energy, carbon and hydrogen for the anaplerotic reactions. **Table 1** shows the relative amounts and times of consumption of the three main sources of mitochondrial substrates for obtaining energy and intermediary metabolites for the growth and maintenance of the body.

Table 1 shows that carbohydrates stores are small and must be constantly replenished by gluconeogenesis in the liver. Amino acids reserves are practically absent and they are constantly formed due to the digestion of food proteins, as well as in anaplerotic reactions in mitochondria. Carbohydrates are too precious to be used for obtaining energy. Much of glucose, particularly at young age, is used for the synthesis of RNA and DNA, purine and pyrimidine nucleotides. Only erythrocytes, which have no mitochondria utilize glucose for obtaining ATP by glycolysis and NADPH for reducing glutathione. There is an old myth that brain consumes only glucose for supporting its energy needs. However, most of the lactate and neuromediators glutamate and γ-aminobutyric acid, which are also used by synaptic mitochondria as energy substrates, are synthesized by the astrocytes from the carbon atoms of fatty acids and for the expense of energy derived during

Source of Energy (Caloric value– kcal/g)	Storage amount (time of consumption)
Carbohydrates:	Total 4–5 grams (20–30 min)
Blood glucose &	100–120 gram (1–3 hrs.)
Glycogen (CV = 3.81)	
Amino acids	Released during catabolism of food, damaged tissue proteins
(CV = 3.12)	and anaplerotic reactions. The content is highly dynamic.
Acyl Fatty Acids	
(CV = 9.3)	Fat (Kilograms) days

Table 1.
It is shown that carbohydrates stores are small and must be constantly replenished by gluconeogenesis in the liver. Amino acids reserves are practically absent and they are constantly formed due to the digestion of food proteins, as well as in anaplerotic reactions in mitochondria. Carbohydrates are too precious to be used for obtaining energy. Much of glucose, particularly at young age, is used for the synthesis of RNA and DNA, purine and pyrimidine nucleotides. Only erythrocytes, which have no mitochondria utilize glucose for obtaining ATP by glycolysis and NADPH for reducing glutathione. There is an old myth that brain consumes only glucose for supporting its energy needs. However, most of the lactate and neuromediators glutamate and γ-aminobutyric acid, which are also used by synaptic mitochondria as energy substrates, are synthesized by the astrocytes from the carbon atoms of fatty acids and for expense of energy derived during β-oxidation of fatty acids. Synaptic mitochondria also gladly oxidize fatty acids in the presence of supporting substrates [85, 87].

β-oxidation of fatty acids. Synaptic mitochondria also gladly oxidize fatty acids in the presence of supporting substrates [85, 87].

The energetic efficiency of β-oxidation of fatty acids in the presence of supporting substrates is the only combination of substrates capable to support the highest rates of oxidative phosphorylation in the heart during maximal physical loads. The efficiency is achieved by the reduction of not only NADH/NAD^+ system in mitochondria, but also by reduction of the membrane pool of ubiquinol/ubiquinone. Therefore, during β-oxidation of fatty acids, electrons enter the respiratory chain not only from Complex I, but mainly through complexes II and III. However, when the energy demands by the organ's functions diminish, the excess of energy in mitochondria may redirect electrons for production of the superoxide radicals, and thus $HO_2^{\bullet}$ [66, 88]. Oxidation by mitochondria of the NAD-dependent substrates cannot provide high rates of ATP and ROS production because NADH-dehydrogenase activity of Complex I is the rate limiting step [141].

Brandt [21] observed that the rate of ROS production may be increased, when mitochondria have abundant supply of substrates and low level of ATP consumption (low functional load), and diminish when consumption of energy is high, or the substrate supply is limiting. This explains why the symptoms of MetS strongly depend on the life style. This is probably the main reason why men start aging faster and earlier then women. At the age of 45–50, many men reduce physical activity, eat too much and abuse alcohol, which dramatically accelerates ROS production.

After menopause, the women's hormonal status becomes closer to that of men, and therefore they also must utilize fatty acids as the main substrates for energy production. At the post-reproductive stage of ontogenesis, we can assume that both men and women have metabolic pattern similar to their distant ancestors, who did not consume a lot of carbohydrates. This may explain the origin of the insulin resistance at MetS. This is not a pathology rather than a new physiological reality due to metabolic reprogramming at the post-reproductive stage. With low insulin sensitivity, most consumed carbohydrates are directed to the synthesis of lipids, which accelerates obesity, first of all visceral obesity. Excessive food consumption plus lower physical and mental activities accelerate production of superoxide radicals, and, thus, perhydroxyl radicals. This accelerates IPLP yielding harmful products, which have proinflammatory activities, cause damages to proteins, cardiolipin and PEA resulting in mitochondrial dysfunctions and accelerating aging.

For a long time, these gradually accumulating various functional disorders and structural damages are not accompanied by specific clinical manifestations. In people predisposed to an earlier aging, the clinical symptoms may be unspecific and look like frailty. With time, the accumulated wear and tear will cause development of clinical symptoms, like acute heart failure, Alzheimer's disease, or something else, and finally death.

Literature show diminished fatty acids oxidation and developments of MetS symptoms in the females without estrogen that can be normalized by administration of estrogen [142, 143]. We do not think that those publications contradict to our conclusions presented in this Chapter, because those experiments have been done on young animals 7–8 weeks old.

17. Conclusions

In this Chapter we have presented evidence that activation of IPLP by hydroperoxyl radical, protonated form of superoxide radical, provides explanation to the slow and inevitable mechanism of aging and resolves many objections against MFRTA in the current paradigms. We also have shown that focusing only on the

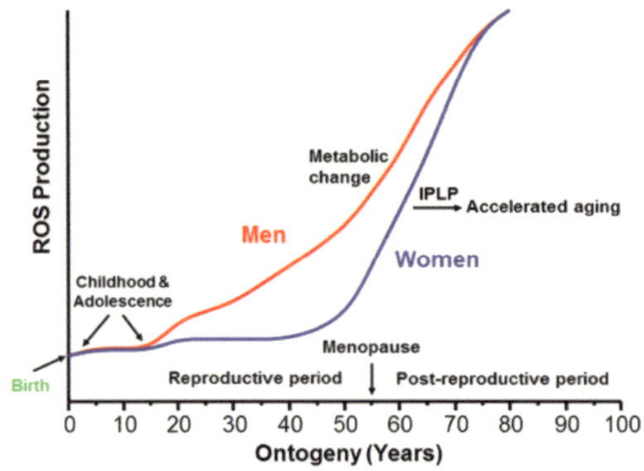

Figure 4.
A schematic presentation of approximate differences between men and women in ROS production during ontogeny. The figure was created based on the data presented in Refs. [111, 112, 116–118, 122, 138].

damages, which accompany aging, is not very helpful, because it gives no answers on why and when aging actually starts, and why women age slower and live longer than men. We have explained the idea that aging is, first of all, the process of development in time, when men and women go through a number of genetically predetermined stages. Because men and women have different biological roles, they also have different metabolic strategies. Fatty acids at all stages of ontogeny are the main substrates for provision of energy and intermediate metabolites for the growth and maintenance. The energetic efficiency of β-oxidation of fatty acids is controlled by the type of mitochondrial metabolites that oxidize simultaneously with fatty acids. However, this results in a significant increase in oxidative stress. We suggest that sex hormones determine the type and quantity of supporting substrates, which result in different rates of energy production and oxidative stress. Women consume more fatty acids with lower efficiency, and thus age at a slower pace. When men and women enter the post-reproductive stage of the ontogeny, the type of metabolism also changes because this last stage of ontogeny is controlled by ancient genes of our distant predecessors. In **Figure 4** we summarized the available information as a scheme, which shows the approximate differences between men and women in ROS production during ontogeny. The metabolic syndrome, which usually begin developing after the age of 45 in men and 55 in women, reflects two main events: the transition to the post-reproductive stage of ontogeny, and the new type of metabolism. Because fatty acids become the major substrates for the energy production in all organs, the rate of ROS production, and, consequently, the rate of aging may increase dramatically. The specific symptoms of the MetS prevailing in particular individuals will depend on the genetic background of their ancestors and the life style.

Acknowledgements

This work was supported by funding from National Institute of Health (R01HL144943).

Author details

Alexander V. Panov[1*], Marina A. Darenskaya[1], Sergey I. Dikalov[2] and Sergey I. Kolesnikov[1]

1 Federal Scientific Center for Family Health and Human Reproduction Problems, Irkutsk, Russian Federation

2 Division of Clinical Pharmacology, Vanderbilt University Medical Center, Nashville, TN, USA

*Address all correspondence to: alexander.panov55@gmail.com

References

[1] Villeponteau B. The heterochromatin loss model of aging. Experimental gerontology. 1997;32(4-5):383-394. DOI: 10.1016/S0531-5565(96)00155-6

[2] Tsurumi A, Li W. Global heterochromatin loss: a unifying theory of aging? Epigenetics. 2012;7(7):680-688. DOI: 10.4161/epi.20540

[3] Fukada SI, Ma Y, Uezumi A. Adult stem cell and mesenchymal progenitor theories of aging. Frontiers in cell and developmental biology. 2014;2:10. DOI: 10.3389/fcell.2014.00010

[4] Brown-Borg HM. Hormonal regulation of longevity in mammals. Ageing research reviews. 2007;6(1):28-45. DOI: 10.1016/j.arr.2007.02.005

[5] Kosmadaki MG, Gilchrest BA. The role of telomeres in skin aging/ photoaging. Micron. 2004;35(3):155-159. DOI: 10.1016/j.micron.2003. 11.002

[6] Kruk PA, Rampino NJ, Bohr VA. DNA damage and repair in telomeres: relation to aging. Proceedings of the National Academy of Sciences. 1995; 92(1):258-262. DOI: 10.1073/ pnas.92.1.258

[7] Ben-Avraham D. Epigenetics of aging. In Longevity Genes, New York: Springer; 2015. p. 179-191. DOI: 10.1007/978-1-4939-2404-2_9

[8] Harman D. Aging: a theory based on free radical and radiation chemistry. J Gerontol. 1956;11:298-300.

[9] Harman D. The biologic clock: the mitochondria? Journal of the American Geriatrics Society. 1972;20(4):145-147. DOI: 10.1111/j.1532-5415.1972.tb00787.x

[10] Harman D. The aging process. Proceedings of the National Academy of Sciences. 1981;78(11):7124-7128. DOI: 10.1073/pnas.78.11.7124

[11] Harman D. Free radical theory of aging: consequences of mitochondrial aging. Age. 1983;6(3):86-94. DOI: 10.1007/BF02432509

[12] Harman D. The free radical theory of aging. Antioxidants and Redox Signaling. 2003;5(5):557-561. DOI: 10.1089/152308603770310202

[13] Harman D. Free radical theory of aging: an update: increasing the functional life span. Annals of the New York academy of sciences. 2006;1067(1):10-21. DOI: 10.1196/ annals.1354.003

[14] Beckman KB, Ames BN. The free radical theory of aging matures. Physiological reviews. 1998;78(2):547-581. DOI: 10.1152/physrev. 1998.78.2.547

[15] Barja G. Updating the mitochondrial free radical theory of aging: an integrated view, key aspects, and confounding concepts. Antioxidants & redox signaling. 2013;19(12):1420-1445. DOI: 10.1089/ars.2012.5148

[16] Barja G. The mitochondrial free radical theory of aging. Prog Mol Biol Transl Sci. 2014;127:1-27. DOI: 10.1016. B978-0-12-394625-6.00001-5

[17] Barja G, Cadenas S, Rojas C, Perez-Campo R, Lopez-Torres M. Low mitochondrial free radical production per unit O2 consumption can explain the simultaneous presence of high longevity and high aerobic metabolic rate in birds. Free radical research. 1994;21(5):317-327. DOI: 10.3109/107157694090 56584

[18] Muller F. The nature and mechanism of superoxide production by the electron transport chain: its relevance to aging. Journal of the American Aging Association. 2000;23(4):227-253. DOI:10.1007/s11357-000-0022-9

[19] Murphy MP, Partridge L. Toward a control theory analysis of aging. Annu. Rev. Biochem. 2008;77:777-798. DOI: 10.1146/annurev.biochem.77.070606.101605

[20] Indo HP, Yen HC, Nakanishi I, Matsumoto KI, Tamura M, Nagano Y, Minamiyama Y. A mitochondrial superoxide theory for oxidative stress diseases and aging. Journal of clinical biochemistry and nutrition. 2015;56(1):1-7. DOI: 10.3164/jcbn.14-42

[21] Brand MD. Mitochondrial generation of superoxide and hydrogen peroxide as the source of mitochondrial redox signaling. Free Radical Biology and Medicine. 2016;100:14-31. DOI: 10.1016/j.freeradbiomed.2016.04.001

[22] Murphy MP. How mitochondria produce reactive oxygen species. Biochemical journal. 2009;417(1):1-13. DOI: 10.1042/BJ20081386

[23] Boveris A, Chance B. The mitochondrial generation of hydrogen peroxide. General properties and effect of hyperbaric oxygen. Biochemical Journal. 1973;134(3):707-716. DOI: 10.1042/bj1340707

[24] Chance B, Sies H, Boveris A. Hydroperoxide metabolism in mammalian organs. Physiological reviews. 1979;59(3):527-605. DOI: 10.1152/physrev.1979. 59.3.527

[25] Wallace DC. Mitochondria and cancer: Warburg addressed. In Cold Spring Harbor symposia on quantitative biology, Cold Spring Harbor Laboratory Press. 2005;70:363-374. DOI: 10.1101/sqb.2005.70.035

[26] Ryzhkova AI, Sazonova MA, Sinyov VV, Galitsyna EV, Chicheva MM, Melnichenko AA, Shkurat TP. Mitochondrial diseases caused by mtDNA mutations: a mini-review. Therapeutics and clinical risk management. 2018;14: 1933-1942. DOI: 10.2147/TCRM.S154863

[27] Volobueva A, Grechko A, Yet SF, Sobenin I, Orekhov A. Changes in mitochondrial genome associated with predisposition to atherosclerosis and related disease. Biomolecules. 2019;9(8):377. DOI: 10.3390/biom9080377

[28] Sequeira A, Martin MV, Rollins B, Moon EA, Bunney WE, Macciardi F, Lupoli S, Smith EN, Kelsoe J, Magnan CN, van Oven M, Baldi P, Wallace DC, Vawter MP. Mitochondrial mutations and polymorphisms in psychiatric disorders. Front Genet. 2012;3:103. DOI: 10.3389/fgene.2012.00103

[29] Tranah GJ, Katzman SM, Lauterjung K, Yaffe K, Manini TM, Kritchevsky S, Newman AB, Harris TB, Cummings SR. Mitochondrial DNA m.3243A > G heteroplasmy affects multiple aging phenotypes and risk of mortality. Sci Rep. 2018;8(1):11887. DOI: 10.1038/s41598-018-30255-6

[30] Pinto M, Moraes CT. Mechanisms linking mtDNA damage and aging. Free Radical Biology and Medicine. 2015;85:250-258. DOI: 10.1016/j.freeradbiomed. 2015.05.005

[31] Szczepanowska K, Trifunovic A. Origins of mtDNA mutations in ageing. Essays in biochemistry. 2017;61(3):325-337. DOI: 10.1042/EBC20160090

[32] DeBalsi KL, Hoff KE, Copeland WC. Role of the mitochondrial DNA replication machinery in mitochondrial DNA mutagenesis, aging and age-related diseases. Ageing research reviews. 2017;33:89-104. DOI: 10.1016/j.arr.2016.04.006

[33] Chocron ES, Munkácsy E, Pickering AM. Cause or casualty: The role of mitochondrial DNA in aging and

age-associated disease. Biochimica et Biophysica Acta (BBA)-Molecular Basis of Disease. 2019;1865(2):285-297. DOI: 10.1016/j.bbadis.2018.09.035

[34] Halliwell B, Gutteridge JM. Oxygen toxicity, oxygen radicals, transition metals and disease. Biochemical journal. 1984;219(1):1-14. DOI: 10.1042/bj21 90001

[35] Brown GC, Borutaite V. There is no evidence that mitochondria are the main source of reactive oxygen species in mammalian cells. Mitochondrion. 2012;12(1):1-4. DOI: 10.1016/j. mito.2011.02.001

[36] Veith A, Moorthy B. Role of cytochrome p450s in the generation and metabolism of reactive oxygen species. Current opinion in toxicology. 2018;7:44-51. DOI: 10.1016/j. cotox.2017.10.003

[37] Battelli MG, Polito L, Bortolotti M, Bolognesi A. Xanthine oxidoreductase-derived reactive species: physiological and pathological effects. Oxidative medicine and cellular longevity. 2016:2016. DOI: 10.1155/2016/3527579

[38] Bonekamp NA, Völkl A, Fahimi HD, Schrader M. Reactive oxygen species and peroxisomes: struggling for balance. Biofactors. 2009;35(4):346-355. DOI: 10.1002/biof.48

[39] Panov AV, Kubalik N, Zinchenko N, Ridings DM, Radoff DA, Hemendinger R, Bonkovsky HL. Metabolic and functional differences between brain and spinal cord mitochondria underlie different predisposition to pathology. American Journal of Physiology-Regulatory, Integrative and Comparative Physiology. 2011;300(4):R844-R854. DOI: 10.1152/ ajpregu.00528. 2010

[40] Lubos E, Loscalzo J, Handy DE. Glutathione peroxidase-1 in health and disease: from molecular mechanisms to therapeutic opportunities. Antioxidants & redox signaling. 2011;15(7):1957-1997. DOI: 10.1089/ars.2010.3586

[41] Vaish S, Gupta D, Mehrotra R, Mehrotra S, Basantani MK. Glutathione S-transferase: a versatile protein family. 3 Biotech. 2020;10(7):1-19. DOI: 10.1007/ s13205-020-02312-3

[42] Xia L, Liu Y, Zhang S, Yang Y, Zhou Z, Tu J. Can Prohibitin 1 be a Safeguard against liver disease? Annals of Hepatology. 2019;18(6):790-795. DOI: 10.1016/ j.aohep.2019.07.012

[43] Ozaki M. Cellular and molecular mechanisms of liver regeneration: Proliferation, growth, death and protection of hepatocytes. In Seminars in Cell & Developmental Biology. Academic Press. 2020;100:62-73. DOI:10.1016/j.semcdb. 2019.10.007

[44] Popper H. General pathology of the liver: light microscopic aspects serving diagnosis and interpretation. In: Seminars in Liver Disease. Thieme Medical Publishers, Inc.; 1986. p. 175-184.

[45] Schmucker DL. Aging and the liver: an update. The Journals of Gerontology Series A: Biological Sciences and Medical Sciences. 1998;53(5):B315-B321. DOI: 10.1093/ gerona/53A.5.B315

[46] Wang Y, Branicky R, Noë A, Hekimi S. Superoxide dismutases: Dual roles in controlling ROS damage and regulating ROS signaling. Journal of Cell Biology. 2018;217(6):1915-1928. DOI: 10.1083/jcb.201708007

[47] DT S, Valentine JS. How super is superoxide. Acc Chem Res. 1981;14:393-400.

[48] Bielski BH, Arudi RL, Sutherland M. A study of the reactivity of HO_2/O_2-with unsaturated fatty acids. J. Biol. Chem. 1983;258:4759-4761.

[49] Pacher P, Beckman JS, Liaudet L. Nitric oxide and peroxynitrite in health and disease. Physiological reviews. 2007;87(1):315-424. DOI: 10.1152/physrev. 00029.2006

[50] Radi R. Oxygen radicals, nitric oxide, and peroxynitrite: Redox pathways in molecular medicine. Proceedings of the National Academy of Sciences. 2018;115(23):5839-5848. DOI: 10.1073/pnas.1804932115

[51] Beckman JS, Koppenol WH. Nitric oxide, superoxide, and peroxynitrite: the good, the bad, and ugly. American Journal of Physiology-cell physiology. 1996;271(5):C1424-C1437. DOI: 10.1152/ajpcell.1996.271.5.C1424

[52] Halliwell B, Gutteridge JM. Free radicals in biology and medicine. USA: Oxford University Press; 2015. 906 p.

[53] Pryor WA, Stanley JP, Blair E, Cullen GB. Autoxidation of Polyunsaturated Fatty Acids: Part I. Effect of Ozone on the Autoxidation of Neat Methyl Linoleate and Methyl Linolenate. Archives of Environmental Health: An International Journal. 1976;31(4):201-210. DOI: 10.1080/00039896.1976.10667220

[54] Pryor WA, Houk KN, Foote CS, Fukuto JM, Ignarro LJ, Squadrito GL, Davies KJ. Free radical biology and medicine: it's a gas, man! American Journal of Physiology-Regulatory, Integrative and Comparative Physiology. 2006;291(3): R491-R511. DOI: 10.1152/ajpregu.00614.2005

[55] Panov AV, Dikalov SI. Mitochondrial Metabolism and the Age-Associated Cardiovascular Diseases. EC Cardiology. 2018;5:750-769.

[56] Sanz A, Pamplona R, Barja G. Is the mitochondrial free radical theory of aging intact? Antioxidants & redox signaling. 2006;8(3-4):582-599. DOI: 10.1089/ars.2006.8.582

[57] Sanz A, Stefanatos RK. The mitochondrial free radical theory of aging: a critical view. Curr. Aging Sci. 2008;1:10-21.

[58] Scialo F, Mallikarjun V, Stefanatos R, Sanz A. Regulation of lifespan by the mitochondrial electron transport chain: reactive oxygen species-dependent and reactive oxygen species-independent mechanisms. Antioxid Redox Signal. 2013;19(16):1953-1969. DOI: 10.1089/ars.2012.4900

[59] Paradies G, Petrosillo G, Paradies V, Ruggiero FM. Role of cardiolipin peroxidation and Ca2+ in mitochondrial dysfunction and disease. Cell Calcium. 2009;45(6):643-650. DOI: 10.1016/j.ceca.2009.03.012

[60] Paradies G, Petrosillo G, Paradies V, Ruggiero FM. Mitochondrial dysfunction in brain aging: role of oxidative stress and cardiolipin. Neurochem Int. 2011;58(4):447-457. DOI: 10.1016/j.neuint.2010.12.016

[61] Shabalina IG, Vyssokikh MY, Gibanova N, Csikasz RI, Edgar D, Hallden-Waldemarson A, Rozhdestvenskaya Z, Bakeeva LE, Vays VB, Pustovidko AV, Skulachev MV, Cannon B, Skulachev VP, Nedergaard J. Improved health-span and lifespan in mtDNA mutator mice treated with the mitochondrially targeted antioxidant SkQ1. Aging (Albany NY). 2017;9(2):315-339. DOI: 10.18632/aging.101174

[62] Stefanova NA, Ershov NI, Maksimova KY, Muraleva NA, Tyumentsev MA, Kolosova NG. The Rat Prefrontal-Cortex Transcriptome: Effects of Aging and Sporadic Alzheimer's Disease-Like Pathology. J Gerontol A Biol Sci Med Sci. 2019;74(1):33-43. DOI: 10.1093/gerona/gly198

[63] De Grey AD. HO2•: the forgotten radical. DNA Cell Biol. 2002;21:251-257. DOI: 10.1089/104454902753759672

[64] Panov A. Mitochondrial production of perhydroxyl radical (HO2•) as inducer of aging and related pathologies. J. Biochem. Biophys. 2017;1(1):105.

[65] Panov A. Perhydroxyl radical (HO2•) as inducer of the isoprostane lipid peroxidation in mitochondria. Mol. Biol. 2018;52:295-305. DOI: 10.1134/S0026 893318020097

[66] Panov AV. A New Look at the Causes of Heart Failure at Old Age. EC Cardiology. 2020;7.2(2020):01-07.

[67] Panov AV, Dikalov SI. Cardiolipin, Perhydroxyl Radicals and Lipid Peroxidation in Mitochondrial Dysfunctions and Aging. Oxidative Medicine and Cellular Longevity. (2020) In press

[68] Bielski BHJ. Reevaluation of the spectral and kinetic properties of HO2• and O2• free radicals. Photochem. Photobiol. 1978;28:645-649. DOI: 10.1111/j.1751-1097.1978.tb06986.x

[69] Gebicki JM, Bielski BHJ. Comparison of the capacities of the perhydroxyl and the superoxide radicals to initiate chain oxidation of linoleic acid. J. Am. Chem. Soc. 1981;103:7020-7022. DOI: 10.1021/ja00413a066

[70] Abner EL, Schmitt FA, Mendiondo MS, Marcum JL, Kryscio RJ. Vitamin E and all-cause mortality: a meta-analysis. Curr. Aging Sci. 2011;4(2):158-170.

[71] Morrow JD, Hill KE, Burk RF, Nammour TM, Badr KF, Roberts LJ. A series of prostaglandin F2-like compounds are produced in vivo in humans by a non-cyclooxygenase, free radical-catalyzed mechanism. Proc. Natl. Acad. Sci. USA. 1990;87:9383-9387. DOI: 10.1073/pnas.87.23.9383

[72] Roberts LJ, Montine TJ, Markesbery WR, Tapper AR, Hardy P, Chemtob S, Dettbarn WD, Morrow JD. Formation of isoprostane-like compounds (neuroprostanes) in vivo from docosahexaenoic acid. J. Biol. Chem. 1988;273: 13605-13612. DOI: 10.1074/jbc.273.22.13605

[73] Morrow JD, Awad JA, Boss HJ, Blair IA, Roberts LJ. Non-cyclooxygenase-derived prostanoids (F2-isoprostanes) are formed in situ on phospholipids. Proc. Natl. Acad. Sci. USA. 1992;89:10721-10725. DOI: 10.1073/pnas.89.22.10721

[74] Montine TJ, Morrow JD. Fatty acid oxidation in the pathogenesis of Alzheimer's disease. Am. J. Pathol. 2005;166:1283-1285. DOI: 10.1016/S0002-9440(10)62347-4

[75] Milne GL, Yin H, Morrow JD. Human biochemistry of the isoprostane pathway. J. Biol. Chem. 2008;283:15533-15537. DOI: 10.1074/jbc.R700047200

[76] Musiek ES, Yin H, Milne GL, Morrow JD. Recent advances in the biochemistry and clinical relevance of the isoprostane pathway. Lipids. 2005;40:987-994. DOI: 10.1007/s11745-005-1460-7

[77] Roberts LJ, Milne GL. Isoprostanes. J. Lipid Res. 2009;50:S219-S223. DOI: 10.1194/jlr.R800037-JLR200

[78] Christie W. Isoprostanes. http://lipidlibrary.aocs.org/Primer/content.cfm? ItemNumber =39314. (2006)

[79] Davies SS. Modulation of protein function by isoketals and levuglandins. Subcel. Biochem. 2008;49:49-70. DOI: 10.1007/978-1-4020-8831-5_2

[80] Montuschi P, Barnes PJ, Roberts LJ. Isoprostanes: markers and mediators of

oxidative stress. FASEB J. 2004;18:1791-1801. DOI: 10.1096/fj.04-2330rev

[81] Brame CJ, Boutaud O, Davies SS, Yang T, Oates JA, Roden D, Roberts LJ. Modification of proteins by isoketal-containing oxidized phospholipids. J. Biol. Chem. 2004;279(14):13447-13451. DOI: 10.1074/jbc.M313349200

[82] Davies SS, Roberts LJ. F2-isoprostanes as an indicator and risk factor for coronary heart disease. Free Rad. Biol. Med. 2011;50:559-566. DOI: 10.1016/j.freeradbiomed.2010.11.023

[83] Anderson AP, Luo X, Russell W, Yin YW. Oxidative damage diminishes mitochondrial DNA polymerase replication fidelity. Nucleic Acids Res. 2020;48(2):817-829. DOI: 10.1093/nar/gkz1018

[84] Quinlan CL, Perevoshchikova IV, Hey-Mogensen M, Orr AL, Brand MD. Sites of reactive oxygen species generation by mitochondria oxidizing different substrates. Redox Biology. 2013;1:304-312. DOI: 10.1016/j.redox.2013.04.005

[85] Panov A, Schonfeld P, Dikalov S, Hemendinger R, Bonkovsky HL, Brooks BR. The Neuromediator Glutamate, through Specific Substrate Interactions, Enhances Mitochondrial ATP Production and Reactive Oxygen Species Generation in Nonsynaptic Brain Mitochondria. J. Biol. Chem. 2009;284:14448-14456. DOI: 10.1074/jbc.M900985200

[86] Panov A. Practical Mitochondriology. Pitfalls and problems in studies of mitochondria with description of mitochondrial functions. Create Space: Amazon-Kindle; 2014. ISBN: 9781483963853.

[87] Panov A, Orynbayeva Z, Vavilin V, Lyakhovich V. Fatty Acids in Energy Metabolism of the Central Nervous System. Review Article. BioMed. Res. International. 2014;2014:22. DOI: 10.1155/2014/472459

[88] Panov AV. Synergistic oxidation of fatty acids, glucose and amino acids metabolites by isolated rat heart mitochondria. EC Cardiology. 2018;5:198-208.

[89] Perevoshchikova IV, Quinlan CL, Orr AL, Gerencser AA, Brand MD. Sites of superoxide and hydrogen peroxide production during fatty acid oxidation in rat skeletal muscle mitochondria. Free Radic. Biol. Med. 2013;61C:298-309. DOI: 10.1016/j.freeradbiomed.2013.04.006

[90] Morris CW. Academic Press Dictionary of Science and Technology. California, San-Diego: Academic Press, Inc.; 1992. 2380 p.

[91] Gould SJ. Ontogeny and Phylogeny. Cambridge, Massachusetts: The Belknap Press of Harvard University Press; 1977.

[92] [Internet]. Available from: http://www.lomonosov-fund.ru/enc/ru/encyclopedia:0132877 [Accessed: 2020-09-15]

[93] López-Otín C, Blasco MA, Partridge L, Serrano M, Kroemer G. The hallmarks of aging. Cell. 2013;153:1194-1217. DOI: 10.1016/j.cell.2013.05.039

[94] Baumann CW, Kwak D, Thompson LV. Sex-specific components of frailty in C57BL/6 mice. Aging (Albany NY). 2019;11(14):5206-5214. DOI: 10.18632/aging.102114

[95] Searle SD, Mitnitski A, Gahbauer EA, Gill TM, Rockwood K. A standard procedure for creating a frailty index. BMC Geriatr. 2008;8:24. DOI: 10.1186/1471-2318-8-24

[96] Fried LP, Ferrucci L, Darer J, Williamson JD, Anderson G. Untangling the concepts of disability, frailty, and

comorbidity: implications for improved targeting and care. J Gerontol A Biol Sci Med Sci. 2004;59:255-263. DOI: 10.1093/gerona/59.3.M255

[97] Panov AV, Golubenko MV. Human Metabolic Syndrome as One of the Last Stages of Postembryonic Ontogenesis. Understanding Human Heart Diseases at Old Age. EC Cardiology 7.8 (2020): 1-47.

[98] Barton NH, Charlesworth B. Why sex and recombination? Science. 1998;281(5385): 1986-1990. DOI: 10.1126/science.281.5385.1986

[99] Hoekstra RF. Evolutionary biology: why sex is good. Nature. 2205;434(7033):571-573. DOI: 10.1038/434571a.

[100] Goddard MR, Godfray HC, Burt A. Sex increases the efficacy of natural selection in experimental yeast populations. Nature. 2005;434(7033):636-640. DOI: 10.1038/nature03405

[101] Hörandl E, Speijer D. How oxygen gave rise to eukaryotic sex. Proc. R. Soc. B. 2018;85:20172706. DOI: 10.1098/rspb.2017.2706

[102] Otto SP, Lenormand T. Resolving the paradox of sex and recombination. Nat Rev Genet. 2002;3(4):252-261. DOI: 10.1038/nrg761

[103] Vina J, Sastre J, Pallardo F, Borras C. Mitochondrial theory of aging: importance to explain why females live longer than males. Antioxid Redox Signal. 2003;5(5):549-556. DOI: 10.1089/152308603770310194

[104] Vina J, Borras C, Gambini J, Sastre J, Pallardo FV. Why females live longer than males? Importance of the upregulation of longevity-associated genes by oestrogenic compounds. FEBS Lett. 2005;579(12):2541-2545. DOI: 10.1016/j.febslet.2005.03.090

[105] Ballard JW, Melvin RG, Miller JT, Katewa SD. Sex differences in survival and mitochondrial bioenergetics during aging in Drosophila. Aging Cell. 2007;6(5):699-708. DOI: 10.1111/j.1474-9726.2007.00331.x

[106] Ali SS, Xiong C, Lucero J, Behrens MM, Dugan LL, Quick KL. Gender differences in free radical homeostasis during aging: shorter-lived female C57BL6 mice have increased oxidative stress. Aging Cell. 2006;5(6):565-574. DOI: 10.1111/j.1474-9726.2006.00252.x

[107] Sengupta P. The Laboratory Rat: Relating Its Age with Human's. Int. J. Prev. Med. 2013;4:624-630.

[108] Demeter E, Sarter M, Lustig C. Rats and humans paying attention: cross-species task development for translational research. Neuropsychology. 2008;22(6):787-799. DOI: 10.1037/a0013712

[109] Zucker I, Beery AK. Males still dominate animal studies. Nature. 2010;465:690. DOI: 10.1038/465690a

[110] Vijay V, Han T, Moland CL, Kwekel JC, Fuscoe JC, Desai VG. Sexual dimorphism in the expression of mitochondria-related genes in rat heart at different ages. PLoS One. 2015;10(1):e0117047. DOI: 10.1371/journal.pone. 0117047

[111] Olivetti G, Giordano G, Corradi D, Melissari M, Lagrasta C, Gambert SR, Anversa P. Gender differences and aging: effects on the human heart. J Am Coll Cardiol. 1995;26:1068-1079. DOI: 10.1016/0735-1097(95)00282-8

[112] Blaak E. Gender differences in fat metabolism. Curr Opin Clin Nutr Metab Care. 2001;4(6):499-502.

[113] Lemieux S, Prud'homme D, Bouchard C, Tremblay A, Després JP. Sex differences in the relation of visceral

adipose tissue accumulation to total body fatness. Am J Clin Nutr 1993;58:463-467. DOI: 10.1093/ajcn/58.4.463

[114] Bjorntorp P. The regulation of adipose tissue distribution in humans. Int J Obes Relat Metab Disord. 1996;20(4):291-302.

[115] Tipton KD. Gender differences in protein metabolism. Curr Opin Clin Nutr Metab Care. 2001;4(6):493-498.

[116] Carter SL, Rennie C, Tarnopolsky MA. Substrate utilization during endurance exercise in men and women after endurance training. Am. J. Physiol. Endocrinol. Metab. 2001;280(6):E898-907. DOI: 10.1152/ajpendo.2001.280.6. E898

[117] Tarnopolsky MA. Gender differences in substrate metabolism during endurance exercise. Can J Appl Physiol. 2000;25(4):312-327. DOI: 10.1139/h00-024

[118] Lamont LS, McCullough AJ, Kalhan SC. Gender differences in the regulation of amino acid metabolism. J. Appl. Physiol. 2003;95:1259-1265. DOI: 10.1152/japplphysiol.01028.2002

[119] Lepers R. Sex Difference in Triathlon Performance. Front. Physiol. 2019;0:973. DOI: 10.3389/fphys.2019.00973

[120] Joyner MJ, Coyle EF. Endurance exercise performance: the physiology of champions. J Physiol. 2008;586(1):35-44. DOI: 10.1113/jphysiol. 2007.143834

[121] Joyner MJ. Physiological limits to endurance exercise performance: influence of sex. J Physiol. 2017;595(9):2949-2954. DOI: 10.1113/jp272268

[122] Ventura-Clapier R, Piquereau J, Garnier A, Mericskay M, Lemaire C, Crozatier B. Gender issues in cardiovascular diseases. Focus on energy metabolism. Biochim Biophys Acta Mol Basis Dis. 2020;1866(6):165722. DOI: 10.1016/j.bbadis.2020.16572

[123] Huang PL. A comprehensive definition for metabolic syndrome. Dis. Model Mech. 2009;2(5-6):231-237. DOI: 10.1242/dmm.001180

[124] Ren J, Pulakat L, Whaley-Connell A, Sowers JR. Mitochondrial biogenesis in the metabolic syndrome and cardiovascular disease. J. Mol. Med. (Berl). 2010;88(10):993-1001. DOI: 10.1007/s00109-010-0663-9

[125] Grundy SM, Cleeman JI. Daniels SR, Donato KA, Eckel RH, Franklin BA, Gordon DJ, Krauss RM, Savage PJ, Smith SC Jr, Spertus JA, Costa F. Diagnosis and management of the metabolic syndrome: an American Heart Association/National Heart, Lung and Blood Institute scientific statement. Circulation. 2005;112:2735-2752. doi: 10.1161/CIRCULATIONAHA.105.169404

[126] Kahn R, Buse J, Ferrannini E, Stern M. The metabolic syndrome: time for a critical appraisal. Joint statement from the American Diabetes Association and the European Association for the Study of Diabetes. Diabetologia. 2005;48:1684-1699. DOI: 10.1007/s00125-005-1876-2

[127] Misra A, Khurana L. The metabolic syndrome in South Asians: epidemiology, determinants, and prevention. Metab. Syndr. Relat. Disord. 2009;7(6):497-514. DOI: 10.1089/met.2009.0024

[128] Reaven GM. Role of insulin resistance in human disease. Diabetes. 1988;37(12):1595-1607. DOI: 10.2337/diab.37.12.1595

[129] Reaven GM. The metabolic syndrome: is this diagnosis necessary?

Am. J. Clin. Nutr. 2006;83:1237-1247. DOI: 10.1093/ajcn/83.6.1237

[130] Björntorp P. Abdominal obesity and the development of noninsulin-dependent diabetes mellitus. Diabetes/Metabolism Reviews. 1988;4(6):615-622. DOI: 10.1002/dmr.5610040607

[131] Vikram NK, Pandey RM, Misra A, Goel K, Gupta N. Factor analysis of the metabolic syndrome components in urban Asian Indian adolescents. Asia Pac. J. Clin. Nutr. 2009;18(2):293-300.

[132] Stančakova A, Laakso M. Genetics of metabolic syndrome. Rev. Endocr. Metab. Disord. 2014;15(4):243-252. DOI: 10.1007/s11154-014-9293-9

[133] Wilmot EG, Edwardson C L, Achana FA, Davies MJ, Gorely T, Gray LJ, Khunti K, Yates T, Biddle SJ. Sedentary time in adults and the association with diabetes, cardiovascular disease and death: systematic review and meta-analysis. Diabetologia. 2012;55(11):2895-2905. DOI: 10.1007/s00125-012-2677-z

[134] Edwardson CL, Gorely T, Davies MJ, Gray LJ, Khunti K, Wilmot EG, Yates T, Biddle SJ. Association of sedentary behaviour with metabolic syndrome: a meta-analysis. PLoS One. 2012;7(4):e34916. DOI: 10.1371/journal. pone.0034916

[135] Sun K, Ren M, Liu D, Wang C, Yang C, Yan L. Alcohol consumption and risk of metabolic syndrome: a meta-analysis of prospective studies. Clin. Nutr. 2014;33(4):596-602. DOI: 10.1016/j.clnu.2013.10.003

[136] Park YW, Zhu S, Palaniappan L, Heshka S, Carnethon MR, Heymsfield SB. The metabolic syndrome: prevalence and associated risk factor findings in the US population from the Third National Health and Nutrition Examination Survey, 1988-1994. Arch. Intern. Med. 2003;163:427-436. DOI:10.1001/archinte.163.4.427

[137] Carr MC. The emergence of the metabolic syndrome. J. Clin. Endocrinol. Metab. 2003;88:2404-2411. DOI: 10.1210/jc.2003-030242

[138] Kim JH, Im JA, Lee DC. The relationship between leukocyte mitochondrial DNA contents and metabolic syndrome in postmenopausal women. Menopause. 2012;19(5):582-587. DOI: 10.1097/gme.0b013e31823a3e46

[139] Baños G, Carbó R, Pérez-Torres I. Arachidonic Acid, Metabolic Syndrome and Alternative Therapeutic Agents. In: Arachidonic Acid: Dietary Sources and General Functions Editors: G.G. Dumancas, B.S. Murdianti, E.A. Lucas © 2013 Nova Science Publishers, Inc. ISBN: 978-1-62257-481-0

[140] Bove RM, Patrick E, Aubin CM, Srivastava G, Schneider JA, Bennett DA, De Jager PL, Chibnik LB. Reproductive period and epigenetic modifications of the oxidative phosphorylation pathway in the human prefrontal cortex. PLoS One. 2018;13(7):e0199073. DOI: 10.1371/journal.pone.0199073

[141] Panov A, Dikalov S, Shalbuyeva N, Hemendinger R, Greenamyre JT, Rosenfeld J. Species- and tissue-specific relationships between mitochondrial permeability transition and generation of ROS in brain and liver mitochondria of rats and mice. Am. J. Physiol. Cell. Physiol. 2007;292(2):C708-C718. DOI: 10.1152/ajpcell.00202.2006

[142] Buniam J, Chukijrungroat N, Khamphaya T, Weerachayaphorn J, Saengsirisuwan V. Estrogen and voluntary exercise attenuate cardiometabolic syndrome and hepatic steatosis in ovariectomized rats fed a high-fat high-fructose diet. Am J Physiol Endocrinol Metab.

2019;316(5):E908-E921. DOI: 10.1152/ajpendo.00466.2018

[143] Oliveira MC, Campos-Shimada LB, Marcal-Natali MR, Ishii-Iwamoto EL, Salgueiro-Pagadigorria CL. A Long-term Estrogen Deficiency in Ovariectomized Mice is Associated with Disturbances in Fatty Acid Oxidation and Oxidative Stress. Rev Bras Ginecol Obstet. 2018;40(5):251-259. DOI: 10.1055/s-0038-1666856.

Section 2

Anesthesia and Pain Management

Chapter 4

Anesthetic Consideration for Geriatric Patients

Somchai Amornyotin

Abstract

The geriatric population experiences significant alterations of numerous organ systems as a result of the aging process. They also have several co-morbidities including hypertension, cardiac disease, diabetes, cerebrovascular disease and renal dysfunction. Geriatric patients are considerably vulnerable and especially sensitive to the stress of trauma, surgery and anesthesia. A high incidence of postoperative complications in this population is observed. Appropriate perioperative care was required for geriatric patients. To date, development in anesthesia and surgical techniques has substantially reduced morbidity and mortality in the geriatric patients. Several anesthetic techniques have been utilized for these patients. However, anesthesia-related mortality in geriatric patients is quiet high. All geriatric patients undergoing surgical procedures require a preprocedural evaluation and preparation, monitoring patients during intraprocedural and postprocedural periods as well as postprocedural management. This chapter highlights the physiological changes, preprocedure assessment and preparation, anesthetic techniques, intraprocedural and postprocedural management in geriatric population.

Keywords: anesthesia, analgesia, geriatric, elderly, management

1. Introduction

The geriatric population is quickly growing and living longer, and this development is estimated to significantly increase surgical demand for both elective and emergent cases. Normally, functional reserve and organ functions are declined in the geriatric patients. Perioperative management of geriatric patients is clearly different and commonly more complex than in younger patients. The consequence of surgery and anesthesia in geriatric patients is directly related to the care they receive during the perioperative practice. However, morbidity and mortality rates after surgery in the geriatric patients are significantly higher than the younger patients. Furthermore, inhospital adverse events and prolonged duration of hospital stay are frequently observed in these patients [1, 2]. Although, age itself is not a disease process but instead serves as a chance for developing age-related diseases. The adverse events could be lessened by appropriate preoperative assessment, proper anesthetic technique and careful postoperative management.

2. Cardiovascular system

Physiologic changes of the vascular system include atherosclerosis and increased arterial wall thickness. In addition, aging leads to decrements in the extent of autonomic control of the cardiovascular system. Aging patients have a reduced cardiac output. Systolic function could be remarkably conserved. However, cardiac responsiveness to adrenergic stimulation is declined. Maximal heart rate and cardiac output also decrease with age [3]. Consequently, baroreflex responses could not completely maintain hemodynamic stability in stressful conditions such as orthostatic hypotension and administration of vasoactive drugs. The functional capability of organs declines and co-existing diseases further contribute to this deterioration. Ischemic heart disease, hypertension, diabetes mellitus and hypercholesterolemia are common in the geriatric patients. Subsequently, autoregulation of blood flow to kidney and brain is reduced. The physiological stress response may be impaired because of decreased autonomic function. The cardiac muscle hypertrophy that develops secondary to the increased late systolic afterload leads to myocardial thickening and diastolic dysfunction. Atrial fibrillation is also common in the geriatric patients. Importantly, age changes both pharmacokinetic and pharmacodynamic aspects of anesthetic agents. Response to induction agents results in exaggerated effect on blood pressure. There is also a reduced response to atropine. Moreover, diminished responses to hypovolemia are supplementary confounded by volatile anesthetics and the sedative drugs that impair baroreflex control mechanisms [1, 3].

3. Respiratory system

Functional capacities of the respiratory system are all reduced in the geriatric patients. Decrease in chest wall compliance and the strength of respiratory muscles, making the lungs more difficult to ventilate and declining in maximum inpiratory and expiratory force. Increased alveolar compliance with collapse of small airways and subsequent alveolar hypoventilation, air trapping leading to ventilation perfusion mismatch. Additionally, collapse of small airways, consequent alveolar hypoventilation, and air trapping may lead to ventilation perfusion mismatch. The residual volume is also increased. Ventilatory response to hypoxemia and hypercapnia are deteriorated in the geriatric patients. Hypoxemia can develop easily. Moreover, the prevalence of chronic obstructive pulmonary disease intensely increases with age [4]. Atelectasis and pulmonary infections are more common in these patients. Administration of premedication could increase the patient's risk for aspiration. Combination of residual effects of anesthetic agents, prolonged effect of neuromuscular blocking drugs and postoperative pain, could significantly contribute to the respiratory complications.

4. Renal system

Aging is accompanying with a steady deterioration in renal function. Reduction of glomerular filtration rate, capability to concentrate urine, and reservation of renal function are noted. Monitoring of urine output during and after major surgery would be regularly performed. Geriatric patients do not require a specific fluid regimen. However, they are less able to achieve hypovolemia or hypervolemia. Though, postoperative renal failure is rare, reduced renal blood flow and decreased nephron mass may increase the risk [5]. Risk factors for acute postoperative renal failure include advanced age, diabetes mellitus, preexisting renal insufficiency, major vascular surgery, and recent exposure to nephrotoxins. Sympathetic stimulation, pain, surgical stress, and the use of vasoconstrictive drugs may induce subclinical renal insufficiency.

5. Nervous system

Aging results in a reduction in nervous tissue mass, neuronal density and concentration of neurotransmitters. A reduction of central nervous system function in the geriatric patients is observed. Autonomic dysfunction is related with impairment of cardiovascular reflexes, hypotension, arrhythmias and delayed gastric emptying. Temperature regulation is abnormally seen with increasing age. There is an increase in disorders of cognitive function, memory loss, and degenerative diseases such as Parkinson's disease in these patients. Dose requirements of local and anesthetic agents are reduced. Postoperative cognitive dysfunction increases with aging. Geriatric patients are sensitive to centrally acting anticholinergic drugs. Regional anesthesia or combined general and regional anesthesia could be favorable [6].

5.1 Pharmacology

The reduction of hepatic and renal functions impacts pharmacokinetic and pharmacodynamic of anesthetic drugs. This might be increased the sensitivity to these drugs. In addition, the decrease in total body water leads to a reduction in the central compartment and increased serum concentration after a bolus administration of a drug. Minimal alveolar concentration declines with age. Geriatric patients are more sensitive to anesthetic agents and normally require smaller doses for the same clinical effect. Long-acting drugs would be continued through out the hospital stay. This effect of aging on pharmacokinetic depends upon the drug is used.

5.2 Nutrition

Poor nutrition status is common in the geriatric patients. A meta-analysis presented that perioperative oral nutritional supplementation had a positive effect on serum total protein and led to fewer complications, but did not have a positive effect on postoperative mortality [7]. Prolonged preoperative fasting should be avoided in this population. The recent study has confirmed that preoperative complete geriatric assessment increases ability to predict patients at a greater risk for morbidity and mortality among the geriatric patients with advanced age or multiple comorbidities.

5.3 Musculoskeletal

All types of degenerative diseases encompass the geriatric patients. This may limit exercise tolerance and makes it difficult to assess their fitness. Epidural and spinal blocks are technically difficult. In addition, the geriatric patients are susceptible to fractures and dislocation. Positioning and pressure points should be well taken before and during the procedure.

6. Preoperative preparation

6.1 Assessment

Preoperative geriatric assessment includes functional physical status, neurocognitive function, systematic evaluation of comorbidities, substance abuse, frailty, nutrition, and medication. A complete history and clinical assessment as well as appropriate laboratory testing is required. However, preoperative evaluation of geriatric patients characteristically is more complex than that of younger patients. Moreover, perioperative functional status could be difficult to evaluate. Aging results in the alterations in physiology that are linked to reduce the functional reserve and ability to compensate for the physiological stress.

Assessment of preoperative mental status is critical as it typically reflects on the postoperative cognitive status. Subsequently, the consumption of multiple medications so classic of the geriatric patients can change homeostatic mechanisms. All geriatric patients must have a preoperative anesthetic evaluation and preparation as well as relevant consultations. The geriatric patient is greater risk for long-term functional compromise after the stress of surgery than the younger patient. In general, geriatric patients with complex medical histories are best appreciated before the surgery to ensure that an appropriate preparation. Multidimensional assessments may help redefine standards for accomplishment of surgery [8].

6.2 Preoperative testing

Generally, routine preoperative testing of geriatric patients is not recommended unless coexisting medical sicknesses are identified or suspected. However, in the geriatric patients, our knowledge is somewhat more limited. Recent studies on routine preoperative testing in geriatric patients are observed. To date, it is not clear whether certain preoperative screening tests have a different profit in the geriatric age group. Routine screening in the geriatric patients does not significantly enhance information obtained from the patient's history. Generally, electrocardiogram is compulsory. A chest film would be decided for patients with acknowledged respiratory diseases and patients with symptomatic cardiorespiratory diseases.

According to guidelines of the American College of Cardiology and the American Heart Association for preoperative cardiac assessment, the patient's activity level is a primary element of the necessity for further evaluation [9]. Major predictors of cardiac risk are unstable coronary diseases, decompensated heart failure, significant arrhythmias and severe valvular disease. In patients with intermediate clinical predictors, the type of surgery and functional status of the patients will have major parts in defining the nature and magnitude of preoperative testing. However, no preoperative cardiovascular testing should be implemented if the results will not change perioperative management. In day case surgery, geriatric patients needed careful planning and proper preoperative assessment and preparation.

7. Anesthetic techniques

The determination of the planned anesthetic technique for surgery in geriatric patients should occur in a multidisciplinary approach. Irrespective of the type of anesthetic techniques, anesthesia should be performed by experienced anesthesiologists who are qualified to accomplish the perioperative care of geriatric patients [10]. Generally, all anesthetic techniques may be applied. The choice of anesthesia is prejudiced by numerous factors such as the patient's medical condition, type and duration of surgery, as well as skill of anesthesiologist and surgeon. To date, there is inadequate evidence to support a single best anesthetic plan for geriatric patients. In a recent review, there might be benefits to selecting regional versus general anesthesia as a primary anesthetic modality in certain patient groups. However, this issue remains controversial due to the quality of the studies and the lack of consideration of the risks of neuraxial blockade in several reports [11, 12]. No differences were detected in postoperative morbidity and mortality, rate of readmission as well as hospitalization costs in geriatric patients undergoing regional anesthesia or general anesthesia (GA) for hip surgery [13].

8. General anesthesia

The judgment to use a general anesthesia in geriatric patients is determined by the type of surgery, and anesthesiologist and surgeon preference. Anesthesia preparation time, start time of surgery, length of surgery, time to sit, and time to walk were shorter in GA. Most general anesthetic agents depress cardiovascular and respiratory function as well as change consciousness. There are several adverse effects that happen in unpredictable, varying proportions of geriatric patients, while the cardiorespiratory adverse effects are dose-related. Oxygen desaturation and hypoxemia happens faster in the geriatric patients. Hence, appropriate preoxygenation is critical.

Alterations in pharmacokinetics and pharmacodynamics in geriatric patients affect considerably with the final action of anesthetic drugs and increase the adverse effects. Advanced age is undoubtedly related with a reduction in median effective dose requirements for all anesthetic agents. In geriatric patients, an induction dose of anesthetic agent is substantially reduced. The titration of admistered drugs is extremely recommended. Ketamine should not be used in the patient with cardiac disease or hypertension. GA might be better in geriatric patients with severe cardiorespiratory diseases. Moreover, dementia increases with age. When GA is applied, the time required for clinical recovery from neuromuscular blockade is obviously increased in geriatric patients for nondepolarizing muscle relaxants. A short or intermediate-acting muscle relaxant is planned when tracheal extubation is needed. Once paralysis is not compulsory, laryngeal mask airway could be performed in the geriatric patients with a low risk of aspiration. Careful perioperative fluid balance is required in the geriatric patients. Consequently, GA in geriatric patients is associated with hypothermia, leading to increased morbidity.

9. Regional anesthesia

Regional anesthesia (RA) may have some benefits over general anesthesia, including less thromboembolic events, confusion and respiratory problems postoperatively. Regional techniques could be utilized as a primary anesthetic modality for surgical anesthesia or could be combined with GA as an adjunctive modality to augment intraoperative and postoperative pain relief. Additionally, RA may diminish the requirement for sedative and analgesic drugs. This technique also preserves spontaneous ventilation and probable decreases postoperative complication following pelvic and orthopedic surgery [14]. However, age-related cardiovascular and sympathetic changes as well as the reduction of cardiovascular reserve may create possibly hazardous consequences. Moreover, the risk of nerve palsies, paresthesias, and other complications are increased in the geriatric population.

Peripheral blocks in the geriatric patients demonstrate satisfactory outcomes without compromising the safety of the airway or risking major hemodynamic effects. However, there are some anatomical changes including weakening of spine and intervertebral disks, fibrosis of intervertebral foramina, and reduction in fat in epidural space in these patients. Local anesthetic spread could enhance in the spinal column, and the dose of epidural medications should be decreased and given more slowly in the geriatric patients. Consequently, metabolism and clearance of local anesthetic agents are also delayed with advanced age. The dose of local anesthetic agents would be decreased for both neuraxial and peripheral nerve blocks. Moreover, geriatric patients are more sensitive to the central effects of opioids and are at enlarged risk of apnea following neuraxial opioid administration. In addition, neuraxial anesthesia-induced hypotension usually occurs in geriatric patients. Antiplatelet medications require several days or weeks to wear off. Therefore, ticlopidine should be stopped for 14 days and clopidogrel for 7 days before neuraxial anesthesia. However, nonsteroidal anti-inflammatory drugs and aspirin could be continued.

10. Intravenous sedation

Intravenous sedation for geriatric patients is a safe and effective technique. Normally, it is utilized for mild and moderate surgical procedures especially in the rediology department and endoscopy unit [15–18]. These procedures are typically short duration and do not create severe pain. The aim of intravenous sedation for geriatric patients is to endorse the patient's safety, to minimize physical distress or pain, to provide analgesia and procedural amnesia as well as to return the patients to their baseline level of consciousness. Usually, geriatric patients are sicker with more co-morbid situations than in the younger patients. All these factors make sedation in this group a challenging task. Old age does not describe the complete indications for giving general anesthesia more habitually.

Geriatric patients have increased response to sedoanalgesic drugs with higher risks for hypoxia, respiratory depression, and apnea. Accurate assessment of the depth of anesthesia contributes to titrating drug administration to the individual patient [19]. Sedoanalgesic drugs including midazolam, fentanyl and propofol are generally used. In my sedation practice, fentanyl, midazolam and/or propofol are frequently used in a combination technique in the geriatric patients [16, 17, 20]. To date, propofol has been shown to be safe and is extensively performed for sedation and anesthesia outside the operating room. Compared to younger patients, geriatric patients may require dose reduction of midazolam and/or propofol. My previous report also confirmed that all adult patients could be discharged to the ward within 60 minutes from the end of endoscopic procedure, and the discharge time was not associated with age, American Society of Anesthesiologists physical status, and the total dose of sedative drugs [21].

11. Monitored anesthesia care

Monitored anesthesia care (MAC) is one of the most common anesthetic techniques. To date, technologic advances in the diagnostic procedures have produced an increased demand for MAC technique. Usually, MAC is suggested for geriatric patients who fear or deny general anesthesia or who are at increased risk because of age or certain concomitant medical situations. Preoperative, intraoperative and postoperative management should be performed as geriatric patients receiving general or regional anesthesia. Importantly, geriatric patients should be monitored properly by experienced personnel who are knowledgeable about pharmacokinetics and pharmacodynamics as well as qualified in airway management and resuscitation. MAC is classically selected for geriatric patients who require supervision of vital signs and administration of sedoanalgesic drugs to supplement local infiltration or regional anesthesia. Moreover, oxygen supplementation is recommended in all geriatric patients.

Medications normally used for MAC include midazolam, propofol, fentanyl, and remifentanil. However, interpatient unpredictability is noticeable with midazolam, and some geriatric patients might be delicately sensitive to its pharmacologic effects. Midazolam reduces the slope of the carbon dioxide response curve, and decreases the ventilatory response to hypoxia. Propofol retains a short context-sensitive half-life and a high plasma clearance that produce a quick awakening when utilized as the sole agent even after a sustained continuous infusion. However, propofol creates a dose-dependent effect in cardiorespiratory system [22]. To avoid undesirable effects, it is critical to decrease the initial doses in the geriatric patients. Remifentanil is an ultrashort-acting drug. Its peak effect occurs within 1-2 minutes after bolus administration [20]. Distribution and metabolism of remifentanil permit for early offset and return of spontaneous ventilation. The dose of remifentanil should be calculated to lean body mass and that geriatric patients require as much as 50%-70% dosage reduction.

12. Intraoperative care

12.1 Fluid management

Generally, fluid management should provide into account the combined effects of aging, anesthetics, analgesics, and anxiolytics on physiology. Appropriate use of intravenous fluids in geriatric patients is essential to avoid unpleasant effects of fluid administration. Insufficient hydration may often quickly deteriorate in organ functions. In high-risk geriatric patients, numerous studies have proven that goal-directed hemodynamic therapy significantly reduced postoperative morbidity and mortality [23, 24]. However, perioperative fluid monitoring is essential. The surgical patients will have been fluid depleted for at least 4-6 hours before. An anesthesiologist must be concerned of the volume status. In addition, fluid balance should be maintained during the procedure.

12.2 Pain management

A proper analgesic plan should be conducted in every geriatric patient before an operation. Many geriatric patients hurt from acute or chronic pain and increasingly apply management for their condition. Depression is common in the geriatric patients and is probable to be faced in the geriatric patient with chronic pain. Therefore, the overall proportion of chronic pain management applications increased in this population. Epidural anesthesia should be intensely considered in geriatric patients, as they offer improved function after abdominal surgery. The overwhelming majority of pain lawsuit in the claims database contained invasive procedures such as blocks and injections. An anesthesiologist should concern any unpredicted motor and/or sensory findings, and should cautiously monitor the geriatric patients for a prolonged time after the neuraxial blockade.

13. Postoperative care

13.1 Oxygen therapy

The geriatric patients are less able to increase and preserve ventilation at high levels. In addition, the responsiveness of central nervous system to hypoxia and hypercarbia is reduced. The reduction of protective reflexes, coughing and swallowing with age can cause recurrent aspirations and pulmonary damage. The greatest incidence of myocardial ischemia is on day 2 or 3 postoperatively. Owing to the abnormalities in gas exchange characteristic of the geriatric patients, it is suggested that they should be transported to the postanesthesia care unit with 2-4 L/min of oxygen via nasal cannula, even after minor ambulatory surgery. Importantly, oxygen therapy and closed monitoring in a high dependancy unit might be required for geriatric patients.

14. Postoperative respiratory complications

The remaining effects of anesthesia could all meaningfully cause to respiratory complications [25]. Postoperative hypoxemia may happen in 20%-60% of geriatric surgical patients. As emphasized previously, geriatric patient has an increased alveolar-arterial gradient, decreased respiratory muscle strength, and diminished hypoxic and hypercarbic drives at baseline. Consequently, there is advanced loss of airway reflexes with age. Apnea and interrupted breathing after administration of narcotics are more common. Risk factors for respiratory complications include atelectasis, pneumonia, and pulmonary thromboembolism, advanced age, poor general health status, current infections, pre-existing cardiorespiratory diseases, hypoalbuminemia, and renal impairment. Supine position during recovery increases transpulmonary shunt [6]. Upper abdomen and intrathoracic procedures in geriatric patients have an independent factor in worsening postoperative hypoxemia and other respiratory complications.

Postoperative pulmonary aspiration in geriatric surgical patients is also an essential issue. Decreased respiratory muscle strength, together with reduced cough and swallowing reflexes may lessen clearance of secretions and increase the risk of pulmonary aspiration in the geriatric patients. This hazard is compounded by the effects of anesthetics, sedatives, and narcotics as well as by interventions such as tracheal intubation, nasogastric tube placement, and upper abdominal or head and neck surgery. An anesthesiologist should to be informed the geriatric patient and family members to this impending hazard and to adjust oral intake postoperatively. Geriatric patients also have a higher incidence of postoperative sleep apnea events. In some geriatric patients, intensive care management is neded.

14.1 Hypothermia

Geriatric patients are more at a higher risk of becoming hypothermic owing to anesthetic induced altered thermoregulatory mechanisms and their low basal metabolic rate. Adverse effects of postoperative hypothermia contain cardiac ischemia, arrhythmias, decreased drug metabolism, increased blood loss, wound infection, and prolonged hospital stay. In geriatric patients, every effort should be done to prevent heat losses. Numerous studies have been revealed that maintaining normothermia decreases cardiac morbidity. Several studies have been accomplished to evaluate the effects of many active or passive warming devices and methods including a forced-air warming blanket or heated humidifier circuit on perioperative hypothermia or shivering in geriatric patients [26, 27].

15. Postoperative pain

Geriatric patients are frequently undertreated for pain. Postoperative pain increases the risk of complications in the geriatric patients. However, pain assessment in this population might be difficult due to cognitive impairment, dementia and aphasia. Insufficient postoperative analgesia may be associated with myocardial ischemia and respiratory failure [6]. However, the geriatric patient is enormously vulnerable to drug interactions and has an enhanced probability of undesirable effects. There is a correlation between postoperative pain and cognitive impairment. Postoperative pain might impair cognition and cognitive impairment could affect with the communication of postoperative pain. Multimodal drug therapy and perioperative regional analgesia could be very effective for perioperative pain management in geriatric patients. In addition, a balanced analgesic technique combining opioids, nonopioids and local anesthetic agents is also suggested.

16. Postoperative cognitive impairment

To identify postoperative cognitive impairment, clinician must be aware of the patient's habitual cognitive status to decide a reasonable assessment of alterations from their individual baseline status. Anesthesia had been concerned as a donating cause of postoperative cognitive impairment in the geriatric patients. Impairments are perceived in mood, memory, behavior, judgment, learning, language and motor function. The previous studies revealed that reduced brain functional reserve made the geriatric patients more likely to develop postoperative cognitive impairment [28]. The contributing factors might be narcotics, sedatives, anticholinergic, infection, anesthetic techniques, pain, sleep deprivation and hospitalization. Postoperative cognitive impairment could be categorized into two main groups: postoperative delirium (POD) and postoperative cognitive dysfunction (POCD). POD and or POCD affects 5-50% of geriatric patients.

Delirium is well-defined as an acute alteration in cognitive function that progresses over a brief period of time lasting for a few days to a few weeks. An incidence of POD is dependent on the type of surgery, patient's preoperative physical and cognitive status, and age of the patient. The overall prevalence of POD in geriatric patients after surgery has been appraised to be 10% [29]. The etiology of delirium is probably multifactorial and may include drug intoxication or withdrawal, drug interaction, anticholinergic agents, metabolic disturbances, hypoxia, abnormal carbon dioxide levels, sepsis, inadequate analgesia, and organic brain diseases. The incidence of POD may be less in outpatients than in hospitalized patients because of ambulatory patients return home postoperatively where suitable stimuli and support are obtainable. A previous systematic review for prevention of POD in geriatric patients scheduled for elective surgery presented that multicomponent interventions, antipsychotics, bispectral index-guidance, and dexmedetomidine treatment could successfully decrease an incidence of POD in geriatric patients undergoing elective non-cardiac surgery [30].

POCD is a syndrome well-defined by a deterioration from baseline in cognitive neuropsychological functioning which could last for months up to 1 year and possibly longer. POCD happens at rates as high as 79% at 7 days, 12.7% at 3 months in non-cardiac surgery patients [31]. The risk factors of POCD are multifactorial and may contain lower preoperative cognitive score, less educated, alcohol abuse, electrolyte abnormalities, type of surgical procedure, drug interactions, hypnotic or alcohol withdrawal, intraoperative events related to the surgical procedures as well as anesthetic agents and depth of anesthesia. Furthermore, physiological and sociological consequences of hospitalization and surgery might have a role. The only risk factor for late POCD was age. No differences between regional and general anesthesia in the incidence of postoperative cognitive impairment are noticed [32]. Interestingly, outpatients may have a superior cognitive outcome than inpatients.

17. Other considerations

Generally, postoperative nausea and vomiting (PONV) and pain are the two most common causes for unpredicted admission after scheduled outpatient surgery. Risk factors for PONV are female gender, previous PONV or motion sickness, nonsmoking status, and opioid use. In addition, geriatric patients experience an increased incidence of conduction abnormalities and bradyarrhythmias including atrial arrhythmias and atrial fibrillation. Transient, subclinical hearing loss is not uncommon after spinal anesthesia [33]. The pathophysiology is supposed to encompass movement of perilymph from the ear into the subarachnoid space as cerebrospinal fluid leaks out. The prevalence rate of mild hearing loss after spinal anesthesia differs inversely with the patient's age. Moreover, geriatric patients are at higher risk for drowsiness, confusion, urinary retention, and adverse drug interactions than the younger patiens. For geriatric outpatients, an escort should stay with the patient for at least 24 hours postoperatively.

18. Conclusion

Geriatric patients are exclusively vulnerable and particularly sensitive to the stresses of hospitalization, anesthesia and surgical procedure. However, age alone does not serve as deterrent for surgical procedures. The care of geriatric patients can be complex and will be a growing task. A balance between physiological and psychological alterations is required in these patients. No anesthetic agent or technique is clearly superior for all conditions or settings. Suitable preoperative, intraoperative and postoperative management is needed of geriatric patients. Additionally, anesthesiologists must have a knowledge of the physiological, pharmocokinetic and pharmacodynamic differences before they utilize their anesthetic techniques.

Conflict of interest

I have no conflict of interest.

Author details

Somchai Amornyotin
Department of Anesthesiology, Faculty of Medicine Siriraj Hospital, Mahidol University, Bangkok, Thailand

*Address all correspondence to: somchai.amo@mahidol.ac.th

References

[1] Amornyotin S. Anesthesia for elderly patients. Analg Resusc Curr Res, 2017, 6 (2), 1000149.

[2] Kim KI, Park KH, Koo KH, Han HS, Kim CH. Comprehensive geriatric assessment can predict postoperative morbidity and mortality in elderly patients undergoing elective surgery. Arch Gerontol Geriatr, 2013, 56 (3), 507-512.

[3] Edelstein SB, Metry JE. Anesthesia considerations for the geriatric patient. Curr Geri Rep, 2017, 6 (3), 115-121.

[4] Incalzi RA, Scarlata S, Pennazza G, Santonico M, Pedone C. Chronic obstructive pulmonary disease in the elderly. Eur J Intern Med, 2014, 25 (4), 320-328.

[5] Novis BK, Roizen MF, Aronson S, Thisted RA. Association of preoperative risk factors with postoperative acute renal failure. Anesth Analg, 1994, 78 (1), 143-149.

[6] Lim BG, Lee IO. Anesthetic management of geriatric patients. Korean J Anesthesiol, 2020, 73 (1), 8-29.

[7] Liu M, Yang J, Yu X, Huang X, Vaidya S, Huang F et al. The role of perioperative oral nutritional supplementation in elderly patients after hip surgery. Clin Interv Aging, 2015, 10, 849-858.

[8] Schlitzkus LL, Melin AA, Johanning JM, Schenarts PJ. Perioperative management of elderly patients. Surg Clin North Am, 2015, 95 (2), 391-415.

[9] Eagle KA, Berger PB, Calkins H, Chaitman BR, Ewy GA, Fleischmann KE et al. ACC/AHA guideline update for perioperative cardiovascular evaluation for noncardiac surgery. J Am Coll Cardiol, 2002, 39 (3), 542-553.

[10] White SM, Altermatt F, Bary J, Ben-David B, Coburn M, Coluzzi F et al. International Fragility Fracture Network Delphi consensus statement on the principles of anesthesia for patients with hip fracture. Anaesthesia, 2018, 73 (7), 863-874.

[11] Guay J, Choi P, Suresh S, Albert N, Kopp S, Pace NL. Neuraxial blockade for the prevention of postoperative mortality and major morbidity: an overview of Cochrane systematic reviews. Cochrane Database Syst Rev, 2014, 1, CD010108.

[12] Nordquist D, Halaszynski TM. Perioperative multimodal anesthesia using regional techniques in the aging surgical patient. Pain Res Treat, 2014, 2014, 902174.

[13] Le-Wendling L, Bihorac A, Baslanti TO, Lucas S, Sadasivan K, Heyman J et al. Regional anesthesia as compared with general anesthesia for surgery in geriatric patients with hip fractures: does it decrease morbidity, mortality, and health care costs? Results of a single-centered study. Pain Med, 2012, 13 (7), 948-956.

[14] Urwin SC, Parker MJ, Griffiths R. General versus regional anaesthesia for hip fracture surgery: a meta-analysis of randomized trials. Br J Anesth, 2000, 84 (4), 450-455.

[15] Amornyotin S, Kachintorn U, Chalayonnawin W, Kongphlay S. Propofol-based deep sedation for endoscopic retrograde cholangiopancreatography procedure in sick elderly patients in a developing country. Ther Clin Risk Manage, 2011, 7, 251-255.

[16] Amornyotin S, Kongphlay S. Propofol-based deep sedation for percutaneous radiofrequency ablation in sick elderly patients with hepatocellular

carcinoma in a developing country. J Anesth Crit Care Open Access, 2017, 8 (3), 00303.

[17] Amornyotin S, Srikureja W, Pausawasdi N, Prakanrattana U, Kachintorn U. Intravenous sedation for gastrointestinal endoscopy in very elderly patients of Thailand. Asian Biomed, 2011, 5 (4), 485-491.

[18] Amornyotin S, Leelakusolvong S, Chalayonnawin W, Kongphlay S. Age-dependent safety analysis of propofol-based deep sedation for ERCP and EUS procedures at an Endoscopy Training Center in a developing country. Clin Exp Gastroenterol, 2012, 5, 123-128.

[19] Amornyotin S. Monitoring for depth of anesthesia: a review. J Biomed Graphics Comput, 2012, 2 (2): 119-127.

[20] Amornyotin S. Sedative and analgesic drugs for gastrointestinal endoscopic procedure. J Gastroenterol Hepatol Res, 2014, 3 (7), 1133-1144.

[21] Amornyotin S, Chalayonnavin V, Kongphlay S. Recovery pattern and home-readiness after gastrointestinal endoscopy. J Med Assoc Thai, 2007, 90 (11), 2352-2358.

[22] Amornyotin S. Sedation-related complications in gastrointestinal endoscopy. World J Gastrointest Endosc, 2013, 5 (11), 527-533.

[23] Hamilton MA, Cecconi M, Rhodes A. A systematic review and mata-analysis on the use of preemptive hemodynamic intervention to improve postoperative outcomes in moderate and high-risk surgical patients. Anesth Analg, 2011, 112 (6), 1392-1402.

[24] Gurgel ST, do Nascimento P. Maintaining tissueperfusion in high-risk surgical patients: a systemic review of randomized clinical trials. Anesth Analg, 2011, 112 (6), 1384-1391.

[25] Jin F, Chung F. Minimizing perioperative adverse events in the elderly. Br J Anesth, 2001, 87 (4), 608-624.

[26] Hong S, Yoo BH, Kim KM, Kim MC, Yon JH, Lee S. The efficacy of warming blanket on reducing intraoperative hypothermia in patients undergoing transurethral resection of bladder tumor under general anesthesia. Anesth Pain Med, 2016, 11 (4), 404-409.

[27] Seo H, Kim K, Oh EA, Moon YJ, Kim YK, Hwang JH. Effect of electrically heated humidifier on intraoperative core body temperature decrease in elderly patients: a prospective observational study. Anesth Pain Med, 2016, 11 (2), 211-216.

[28] Strom C, Rasmussen LS. Challenges in anaesthesia for elderly. Singapore Dent J, 2014, 35, 23-29.

[29] Rasmussen LS, Moller JT. Central nervous system dysfunction after anesthesia in the geriatric patient. Anesthesiol Clin North Am, 2000, 18 (1), 59-70.

[30] Janssen TL, Alberts AR, Hooft L, Mattace-Raso F, Mosk CA, van der Laan L. Prevention of postoperative delirium in elderly patients planned for elective surgery: systematic review and meta-analysis. Clin Interv Aging, 2019, 14, 1095-1117.

[31] Berger M, Nadler JW, Browndyke J, Terrando N, Ponnusamy V, Cohen HJ et al. Postoperative cognitive dysfunction: minding the gaps in our knowledge of a common postoperative complication in the elderly. Anesthesiol Clin, 2015, 33 (3), 517-550.

[32] Rasmussen LS, Johnson T, Kuipers HM, Kristensen D, Siersma VD, Vila P et al. Does anesthesia cause postoperative cognitive dysfunction? A randomized study of regional versus

general anesthesia in 438 elderly patients. Acta Anesthesiol Scand, 2003, 47 (3), 260-266.

[33] Gultekin S, Ozcan S. Does hearing loss after spinal anesthesia differ between young and elderly patients? Anesth Analg, 2002, 94 (5), 1318-1320.

Chapter 5

Pain Management in Older Persons

Dabota Yvonne Buowari

Abstract

Pain is a common symptom in the elderly and it is problematic and distressful especially if the polder person is dependent on a caregiver. Pain keeps the sufferer uncomfortable and can affect the person from carrying out daily activities and tasks especially activities of daily living. Pain in the older person may be acute or chronic. Some of the causes of pain in the elderly are neuralgia, musculoskeletal dysfunction especially osteoarthritis, emotional and mental problems, cancer and several other causes. The assessment of pain in the elderly is done using validated pain assessment tools such as the visual analogue scale, verbal rating scales, numeric rating scales, McGill pain assessment questionnaire, pain attitudes, brief pain inventory, and geriatric pain measure. Management of pain in older persons involves non-pharmacological and pharmacological methods. There are some barriers and challenges of pain management in the elderly and also consequences when pain is not properly managed or not managed at all in an older person.

Keywords: older person, pain, non-pharmacological management, opioids, nursing home

1. Introduction

The numbers of older persons are increasing worldwide; which means there will also be an increase in their health needs [1–13]. Sometimes health issues concerning older persons are neglected [14]. The aging process affected by several factors. Older persons may have more than one disease leading to comorbidities as well as chronic pain [14–18]. Generally pain is a common complaint in senior citizens but it is not part of the aging process as pain in the elderly is underreported and under treated [9, 13, 15, 17, 19]. Pain management in older persons is problematic due to the various changes associated with the aging process that occur in the different body organs and systems [10]. The perception of pain is beneficial for survival [15]. Pain management is an important aspect of healthcare [20]. The rudiments of effective pain management includes close monitoring for adverse effects, regular assessment of the pain using various validated pain assessment tools and adjustment of the dose of analgesics administered to the corresponding response. Any pain causing physical and psychosocial functionality problems should be regarded as a significant health problem [15]. Pain is the most common reason why an older person will consult a physician [21].

2. What is pain?

Everyone feels pain though some researchers argue that neonates do not feel pain. The word pain is derived from the Greek word, which means penalty in Greek [20]. The taxonomy of the International Association for the Study of Pain (IASP) defines pain as 'an unpleasant sensory and emotional experience associated with actual or potential tissue damage or described in terms of such damage [20, 22–24]. Pain is a complex phenomenon characterized by a sensory and emotional experience that is unpleasant [25–27] and it is also distressing [28]. Pain is the most common symptom complained by the elderly [29]. Older people tend to underreport pain due to several barriers and challenges such as cultural beliefs and ageism [29]. Pain management is generally under diagnosed, overlooked and undertreated in older adults [15, 27, 30]. Pain is a subjective personal experience known only by the sufferer [30].

3. Prevalence of pain in older persons

The prevalence of pain in the older persons varies, pain is prevalent in older persons and this increases with age [9, 31, 32]. The knowledge of the prevalence of pain in the oldest old is scarce [33]. Several studies have been conducted on pain in older persons. Many reports suggest that the incidence of pain in senior citizens is about 50% in older adults living in the community and about 80% in older persons who are resident in nursing homes [17, 21, 25]. The pain is of significant intensity in 19% of older persons.

4. Types of pain

Pain can be classified as acute or chronic pain depending on its duration. It can also be classified depending on the cause of the pain if it is nociceptive pain that is visceral or somatic origin or neuropathic pain. The prevalence of acute pain in the elderly does not change with aging while that of chronic pain increases with aging [29]. Acute pain is usually a symptom of an illness or injury while chronic pain may be a pointer to specific health problems, as the factors leading to chronic pain may not be identified or eradicated all the time [29].

Chronic pain is now also known as recurrent or persistent pain. Chronic pain occurs for a prolong period of time usually more than three months [21] which may or may not be associated with a well-defined disease process [34], and it is an important health problem in the elderly [24, 34, 35]. Chronic pain is prevalent in the elderly [36, 37]. The clinical manifestations of persistent pain the older persons are often complex and multifactorial [26].

Acute pain can be defined as pain that is of distinct onset, there is an obvious cause and also of a short duration, it indicates acute injury or disease [21]. Persistent pain is common among residents of nursing homes.

5. Causes of pain in older persons

There are several causes of pain in older persons.

1. Pain in the lower extremities for instance can be caused by osteoarthritis which could lead to falls [10, 21, 38]. Osteoarthritis is one of the commonest causes

of joint pain and disability in the elderly hence the goal of its treatment is to reduce its symptoms and prevent disability [21].

2. Low back pain, this may be caused by arthritis, muscular and neurological changes associated with aging [10, 24, 29, 31, 39].

3. Joint arthrosis

4. Depression

5. Intestinal diverticulosis

6. Night time leg pain [26]

7. Spinal cord stenosis [29]

8. Myofascial pain [29]

9. Fibromyalgia [29]

10. Post herpetic neuralgia [29]

11. Post stroke pain syndrome [29]

12. Diabetic peripheral neuropathy [29]

13. Cancer [29]

14. Complications related to gait abnormalities, accidents and polypharmacy [9].

6. Assessment of pain in older persons

There are various ways of assessing pain in older persons and this is challenging for various reasons such as those with diminished cognitive ability, dementia, disorders in communication, and cultural barriers [13, 19, 21, 30, 31, 36, 40, 41]. The first step in an effective pain management is assessment of the pain [31]. Assessment of pain in older persons should include the assessment of the older person functional abilities [10, 42] and it requires a multidisciplinary approach for making a diagnosis. This includes understanding the atypical presentations of pain in older persons including its pathophysiology, the physiological changes associated with aging, common pain presentations and the use of validated pain assessment tools [11, 19, 36]. Self-reporting is the best method of assessing pain and there is a wide range of self-report scales as it provides the most accurate and reliable information [36, 43].

There are many validated pain assessment tools that can be used in the assessment of pain in older persons while each of the tools have its merits and demerits as no single tool will be useful for every patient [39, 43]. Commonly used scales in the assessment of pain in older persons are the visual analogue scales, verbal rating scales, numeric rating scales, McGill pain assessment questionnaire, pain attitudes, brief pain inventory and geriatric pain measure [33, 40, 43]. There may be other medical signs and symptoms that can make the pain assessment difficult [13]. Polypharmacy increases sensitivity to analgesics [35]. Sometimes elderly persons find it difficult using self – report pain scales correctly [38, 43].

7. Treatment of pain in older persons

The management of pain in the elderly can be challenging [14, 15, 35, 42], proper assessment of the pain is very important for its management [44]. Pain management in older persons requires a multidisciplinary approach with the use of non-pharmacological techniques and pharmacological agents that is analgesics and adjuvants [9, 13, 15, 19, 21, 37, 45]. The approach to pain management in older persons differs from that of younger person's [26, 31, 37]. The multidisciplinary approach to pain management in the elderly addresses both the medical and psychosocial requirements of the older person and this involves pharmacotherapy, psychological support and sometimes physical rehabilitation [9, 10, 31] all aimed at the reduction of the pain and improvement of the quality of life [15, 45]. History taking is done; if there is cognitive impairment history may be taken from the caregiver [42]. Older persons cope with pain better than younger people as some people believe that pain is part of the aging process [39].

7.1 Non-pharmacological treatment of pain in older persons

There are many forms of non-pharmacological mode of pain management in older persons, this includes:

1. Exercise, this helps to maintain movement hence it helps the older persons to be active, retain muscle tone and have a greater social interaction [15, 21, 38].

2. Weight reduction [15]

3. Massage [45]

4. Electrotherapy for example transcutaneous electrical nerve stimulation (TENS) [21].

5. Acupuncture, this involves the insertion of special acupuncture needles into designated acupuncture points that are then stimulated with either electrical current or manual manipulation [21].

7.2 Pharmacological treatment of pain older persons

The pharmacological management of pain in the elderly involves the use of the three step World Health Organization analgesics ladder, which is an accepted pain plan universally [21, 36, 46]. The pharmacological management of pain in older persons also involves taking into consideration any existent comorbidity and medications taken for other illnesses to avoid drug-drug interactions and side effects [13, 29, 31, 34]. As in the use or administration of any therapeutic agent, older persons are at risk of adverse reactions [13, 15, 31, 38]. Effective pharmacological treatment of pain involves proper assessment of the pain [26]. The physiologic changes associated with aging affect the pharmacokinetics and pharmacodynamics of drugs in the elderly [36]. Multimodality is required which involves the use of different drugs [13, 47]. Traditionally, analgesics are classified into three groups' namely peripheral analgesics such as acetaminophen; non-steroidal anti-inflammatory drugs (NSAIDs) and opioids.

1. **Acetaminophen:** The pharmacological management of pain in the elderly involves the use of acetaminophen marketed in most countries as paracetamol.

Acetaminophen is the commonly used analgesic [10, 36, 44]. It is used in the first step of the pain management ladder of the World Health Organization [10]. The general approach in pain management in the elderly is to start with a non-opioid such as acetaminophen and non-steroidal anti-inflammatory drugs and then use opioids for severe pain [13].

2. **Non-Steroidal Anti-Inflammatory Drugs (NSAIDs)**: These are non-opioid analgesic agents example of NSAIDs are ibuprofen, piroxicam, diclofenac, ketoprofen, etc. One of the adverse effects of NSAIDs is irritation of the lining of the gastrointestinal tract which can lead to hemorrhage therefore it is not taken in an empty stomach and it is administered with caution in patients with peptic ulcer disease. Prolong use of NSAID generally should be avoided in older persons due to association with gastrointestinal bleeding and renal dysfunction [13].

3. **Opioids:** Opioids is used in the management of severe pain both acute and chronic pain, also used in the management of different types of pain such as nociceptic and neuropathic pain [13, 32]. Several factors affect the pharmacokinetics and pharmacodynamics of opioids such as changes associated with the normal aging process as there is a natural decline in the functions of organs and comorbidities are common in older persons [38, 47]. One of the side effects of opioids especially in senior citizens is respiratory depression [48]. Adverse effects on the central nervous system and others are the same for the general population. There is greater risk of side effects in older persons [36]; one of the feared adverse effects of the use of opioids in the elderly is the risk of falls [38]. Therefore management of pain in older persons should include the physician's experience as fear of the adverse effects frequently hinders prescribing analgesics for older persons [26, 38].

4. **Adjuvants Therapy**: Adjuvants used in the treatment of pain in older persons are tricyclic anti-depressants, topical local anesthetics such as topical lignocaine (lignocaine patch), anti-epileptics hypnotics, anxiolytics and antipsychotics [33, 44].

7.3 Barriers and challenges of pain management in older persons

There are many barriers and challenges to the management of pain in older persons [9, 14, 37, 48]. Pain poses a challenge for both senior citizens and their caregivers [13, 37, 38, 42].

1. Older persons sometimes may be reluctant to report pain hence the pain is not assessed at all and not treated properly or sometimes the pain is diagnosed and treated late [9–11, 13, 15, 16, 19, 31, 35–37, 40, 42, 48, 49].

2. Older persons generally under report pain and therefore it is under treated [13, 15, 19, 21, 26, 31, 33, 36, 42–44].

3. Changes associated with aging such as the pharmacokinetics and pharmacodynamics of drugs and other physiologic changes of the aging process [9, 13, 31, 32, 37].

4. Cultural and religious beliefs that pain is part of the aging process [9, 10, 13, 21, 32, 35, 40].

5. Fear of the manifestation of side effects of opiates which is common in the older persons especially as the older persons is prone to comorbidity [13, 21, 25, 26, 32, 36, 37].

6. Changes in the perception of pain in older persons such as when there is cognitive impairment, dementia, sensory impairment, inability to communicate well, depression, functional impairment, delirium [9, 14, 15, 19, 21, 25, 26, 30, 31, 33, 36, 38, 40, 41, 43, 44]. Depression can alter the perception of pain and also the ability to cope with it [36].

7. Fear of falls and addiction from the administration of opioids [38].

8. Polypharmacy [13, 37].

9. Ageism.

8. Consequences of untreated pain in older persons

There are several effects if pain is not adequately or improperly treated in the older persons, these include:

1. Problems with sleep such as inability to initiate or maintain sleep [49].

2. Problems with mood with the risk of depression and social isolation [19, 43, 49].

3. Interference with the activities of daily living [35].

4. Untreated pain in older persons interferes with all aspects of the older person's life, physical, psychological, social and this can lead to poor quality of life [10, 19, 21, 31, 35, 37, 39].

9. Post-operative pain management in older persons

There has been an increase in the incidence of older persons requiring surgical interventions which it requires proper and adequate pain management after the surgery [38]. Adequate perioperative and post-operative pain management in older persons reduces the risk of post-operative delirium [38]. Use of regional anesthesia reduces postoperative complications and improves post-operative pain control [41, 50]. Multimodal drug therapy should be instituted as it has the advantage of minimizing both the dosages and side effects of any single agent [38, 41, 50].

10. Pain management in nursing homes

Pain is common among residents of institutionalized homes [21, 48]; this presents multifaceted challenges for healthcare practitioners [27]. It provokes a significant challenge to the nursing home caregivers in terms of their ability to provide adequate treatment [48]. Generally patients residing in nursing homes are more frail that other older persons living in the community [48].

11. Conclusion

Pain is common in older persons and may be caused by a variety of disease states. There are many challenges in managing pain in older persons when the pain is not adequately or properly treated, it can lead to some consequences such as sleep disturbance and changes in mood.

Conflict of interest

I have no conflict of interest.

Author details

Dabota Yvonne Buowari
Department of Accident and Emergency, University of Port Harcourt Teaching Hospital, Port Harcourt, Nigeria

*Address all correspondence to: dabotabuowari@yahoo.com

References

[1] Bigala P, Ayiga N. Prevalence and predictors of elder abuse in Mafikeng local municipality in South Africa. Afr Pop Stud, 2014, 28 (1), 463-474.

[2] Amaike B, Bammeke F. Gender differences in seniors preferences and expectations of home care in Lagos State, Nigeria. J Ag Emerg Econ, 2014, 4 (2), 4-31.

[3] Abiodum MG, Adekeye OA, Iruonagbe TC. Counselling services for remediating the biophysical challenges of aged in Nigeria. J Funct Manag, 2011, 3 (1), 89-98.

[4] Micheal SN, Anyebe EE, Danyuma A, Munir AS, Afiniki BS. Public awareness and perception on care for the elder among Funtua residents in Katsina State, North-West, Nigeria. World J Prev Med, 2016, 4 (1), 20-24.

[5] Okoye UO. Family care-giving for ageing parents in Nigeria: gender differences cultural imperatives and the role of education. Inter J Educ Ageing, 2012, 2 (2), 139-154.

[6] Ekot MO. Selected demographic variables and elder abuse in Akwa-Ibom State, Nigeria. Inter J Acad Res Bus Soc Sci, 2016, 6 (2), 1-15, www.hrmars.com assessed April 2018.

[7] Uzobo E, Dawodu OA. Ageing and health: a comparative study of rural and urban aged health status in Bayelsa State, Nigeria. Europ Sci J, 2015, 16 (14), 258-273.

[8] Kurura VP. Issues in geriatric anaesthesia. SAARC J Anaesth, 2008, 1 (1), 49.

[9] Kaye AD, Baluch A, Scott JT. Pain management in the elderly population: a review. Ochsner J, 2010, 10, 179-187.

[10] Jones MR, Ehrhardt KP, Ripoll JG, Sharma B, Padnos IW, Kaye RJ et al. Pain the elderly. Curr Pain Headache Rep, 2016, 20, 1-9.

[11] Kress H, Ahlbeck K, Aldingteingon D, Alon E, Coaccioli S, Coluzzi F et al. Manag chronic pain in elderly patients requires a CHANGE of approach. Curr Med Res Opin, 2014, 30 (6), 1153-1164.

[12] Sijuwade PO. Elderly care by family members: abandonment, abuse and neglect. Soc Sci J, 2008, 3 (8), 542-547.

[13] Cavalieri TA. Management of pain in older adults. J Am Osteopath Assoc, 2005, 105, (3-Suppl), 125-175.

[14] Thor H, Jacob M, Christopher V. Acute postoperative pain management in the older patient. Ag Health, 2011, 7 (6), 813-828.

[15] Pateinakis P, Amygdalas S, Pateinaki M, Pyrpasepaulou A. Chronic pain in the elderly. OA Elderly Med, 2013, 1, (1), 4

[16] Keefe FT, Porter L, Somers T, Shelby R, Wiren AV. Psychological interventions for managing pain in older adults: outcomes and clinical implications. Brit J Anaesth, 2013, 111 (1), 41-45.

[17] Schofield P. Pain management in old adults. Med. 2017, 102 (9), 481-485.

[18] Baker TA, Clay DJ, Johnson-Lawrence V, Minahan JA, Mingo CA, Thorpe J, Ovalle F, Crowe M. Associationofmultiplechronicconditions and pain among older black and white adults with diabetes mellitus, BMC Geriat, 2017, 17, 255, 1-9.

[19] Cavelieri TA. Pain management in the elderly. JAOA, 2002, 102 (9), 481-485.

[20] Kumar KH, Elavarasi P. Definition of pain and classification of pain

disorders. J Adv Clin Res Insights, 2016, 3, 87-90.

[21] Benjamin DG. Pain management in elderly: a challenge to practicing clinicians. IJRCI, 2015, 3 (51), SR1, 1-9.

[22] Rajagopal MR. Pain - Basic Considerations. Indian J Anaesth, 2016, 50 (5), 331-334.

[23] Bonica JJ. International association for the study of pain. Definition, the need of a taxonomy. I Pain, 1979, 6 (3), 247-80.

[24] Scherer M, Hansen H, Gensichen J, Mergenthal K, Riedel-Heller S, Weyerer S, Maier W et al. Association between multimorbidity patterns and chronic pain in elderly primary care patients: a cross – sectional observation study. BMC Family Pract, 2010, 17168, 1-8.

[25] Torvik K, Norditug B, Brenne IK, Rognstad M. Pain assessment strategies in home care and nursing homes in mid-Norway: a cross –sectional survey. Pain Manag Nurs, 2015, 16 (4), 602-608.

[26] American Geriatrics Society. Panel on the pharmacological management of persistent pain in older persons. JAGS, 2009, 57, 1331-1346.

[27] Russell TL, Madsen RW, Flesner M, Rantz MI. Pain management in nursing homes: what do quality measure scores tell us? J Gerontol Nurs, 2010, 36, (12), 49-56.

[28] Williams AC, Craig KD. Updating the definition of pain. Pain, 2016, 2420-2423.

[29] Iliaz R, Ozturk GB, Akpinar TS, Tufan A, Sarihan I, Erten N et al. Approach to pain in the elderly. Geron Geriat Res, 2013, 2 (3), doi: 10.4172/2167-7182_1000125

[30] Royal College of Physicians, British Geriatrics Society and British Pain Society. The assessment of pain in older people: national guidelines. Concise Guidance of Good Practice Series, No 8, London, RCP, 2007.

[31] Bruckenthal P, Reid MC, Reisner L. Special issues in the management of chronic pain in older adults. Pain Med, 2009, 10 (52), 67-78.

[32] Chau DL, Walker V, Pai L, Cho LM. Opiates and elderly: use and side effects. Clin Interv Ag, 2008, 3 (2), 273-278.

[33] Schofield P. Assessment and management of pain in older adults: current perspectives and future directors. Scottish Univ Med J, 2014.

[34] Brochet B, Michel P, Barberger-Gateau P, Dartigues J. Population - based study of pain in elderly people: a descriptive survey. Age Ageing, 1998, 27, 279-284.

[35] Dewar A. Assessment and management of chronic pain in the older person living in the community. Austral J Adv Nurs, 2006, 24 (1), 33-38.

[36] Tracy B, Morrison RS. Pain management in older adults. Clin Therap, 2013, 35 (11), 1659-1668.

[37] Fine PG. Treatment guidelines for the pharmacological management of pain in older persons. Pain Med, 2012, 13, 556-566.

[38] Burgess FW, Burgess TA. Pain management in the elderly surgical patient. Med Health, 2008, 91, (1), 11-14.

[39] Rudy T, Weiner DK, Lieber SJ, Slaboda J, Boston JI. The impact of chronic low back pain on older adults, a comparative study of patients and controls. Pain, 2007, 131, 293-301.

[40] Repka I, Puto G. Chronic pain in the elderly over the age of 65 – a review of selected research tools. J Pub Health Nurs Med Rescue, 2016, 4, 12-16.

[41] Halaszynski TM. Perioperative pain management in the elderly surgical patient. Univ J Med Sci, 2013, 1 (2), 36-49.

[42] Hix MD. Pain management in elderly patients. J Pharm Pract, 2007, 20 (1), 49-63.

[43] Guerriero F, Sugarlata C, Maurizi N, Francis M, Rollone M, Carbone M, Rondanelli M, Perna S, Ricevuti G. Pain management in dementia: so far, not so good. JGG, 2016, 64, 31-39.

[44] Husebo BS, Kunz M, Achterberg WP, Lobbezoo E, Kappeser J, Tudose C, Strand LI et al. Pain assessment and treatment challenges in patients with dementia. Z Neuropsy, 2012, 23, (4), 237-248.

[45] Bruckenthal P, D'Arcy IM. Assessment and management of pain in older adults: a review of the basics topics. Adv Pract Nurs J, 2007, 7 (1).

[46] Betteli G. Anaesthesia for the elderly outpatient: preoperative assessment and evaluation, anaesthetic technique and postoperative pain management. Curr Opin Anaesth, 2010, 23, 726-731.

[47] Malec M, Shega JW. Pain management in the elderly. Med Clin N Am, 2015, 99, 337-350.

[48] Reiman M. The problem of pain management in nursing homes. P & T, 2007, 2007, 32 (9), 494-495.

[49] Molton IR, Terrill AL. Overview of persistent pain in older adults. Amer Psych, 2014, 69 (2), 197-207.

[50] Dervishi A, Zallari K. Post-operative pain management in elderly patients. Inter J Sci Res, 2015, 4 (10), 20-23, www.ijsr.net assessed April 2018.

Section 3

Clinical Implication

Chapter 6

Importance of Geriatric Health Care in India during Covid 19 Pandemic

Kaushik Nag, Nabarun Karmakar and Anjan Datta

Abstract

World is facing a dual challenge of deadly Covid 19 pandemic and economic instability with its best health care facility and advanced science & technology. We need to support and protect our physically and economically vulnerable population like geriatric or elderly people during this difficult time. India has nearly 120 million elderly people with various physical, mental, social, economic, and spiritual problems. Ministry of health has created geriatric centers and geriatric clinics in most of the states. Routine care clinics cannot handle the burden of geriatric population to address their co-morbidities. Rapid training of healthcare professionals of various disciplines in geriatric care, home nursing is now of utmost importance. Government must provide financial support to nongovernmental organizations (NGOs) and other agencies for helping geriatric population by providing affordable health care.

Keywords: Health care, aged, Covid 19, pandemic, India, Geriatric, vulnerable population

1. Introduction

India has developed tremendously in providing health care delivery to the beneficiaries in many folds but not sufficient enough to fulfill the need of its huge population of more than 130 crores. Still we are lacking behind in meeting the health needs of our vulnerable population like elderly, pregnant mother etc. It may be due to lack of adequate number of manpower like doctors, nurses, paramedics, laboratory technician etc., sufficient fund allocated for health in budget and proper health infrastructure development.

Population aging is an inevitable and irreversible process due to improvements in health and medical care. With advancement in medical science and increased life expectancy, elderly population (60 years and above) is growing faster than young population globally [1].

The corona virus disease (COVID-19) pandemic has brought about unprecedented fear and uncertainty, especially among elderly population. The elderly population depends on social connection more than other generations and they are deprived of this socialism due to sudden pandemic and subsequent lockdown in the world. India is also practicing nation-wide lock down and advising social distancing measures to prevent the spread of this infectious disease among vulnerable populations like children, pregnant women and older people (more than 65 years). It has been seen, with aging immune system becomes weak and thus elderly are more prone to develop infectious diseases compared to younger generation. Geriatric populations are more affected with non communicable diseases like diabetes mellitus, hypertension, heart diseases, kidney diseases, chronic obstructive pulmonary diseases (COPD), cancer etc. Recoveries are usually slower and complication arises rapidly in older people compared to adults. They face anxiety and depression simultaneously due to their loneliness and burden of household expenditures, routine health checkups. For millions of elderly, COVID-19 has amplified their already-existing anxieties and turns them into panic mood [2].

The elderly constitutes about 11.5% of the total population of seven billion globally. This proportion of elderly is projected to be double (22%) by 2050 and it will be more than children below fifteen years of age. The proportion of the elderly will increase from 22.4% (as on 2012) to 31.9% in 2050 in developed countries. The proportion of the elderly is projected to be below 11% in least developed countries by 2050. The rapid aging of developing countries is not followed by the increase in personal incomes of that country. The proportion of the elderly is expected to double up from 10.5% to 22.4% in Asia during 2012–2050. Three countries in Asia, Japan (41.5%), South Korea (38.9%), China (34%) predicted to have the highest proportions of the elderly population in the region by 2050. The South Asian Association for Regional Cooperation (SAARC) countries, are likely to have only about 21% elderly population by 2050. The proportion of the elderly in India has been increasing at an increasing rate in recent years and the trend is likely to continue in the coming decades. The elderly population accounted for 7.4% of the total population in 2001, 8.6% in 2011 and has been projected to increase to 19% by the year 2050 in India. It is predicted that, the elderly will constitute about 34% of the total population in the country by the end of the 21st century. Therefore, relatively young India today will turn into a rapidly progressing aging society in near future. The sex ratio of the elderly has increased from 938 women to 1,000 men in 1971 to 1,033 in 2011 and is projected to increase to 1,060 by 2026 given the insignificant decline in mortality among males particularly during adult and older years [1, 3, 4].

2. Geriatric problems in India

2.1 Health problems of elderly

In India, the elderly people suffer from dual medical problems, i.e. both communicable as well as non-communicable diseases. It is estimated that one out of two elderly in India suffers from at least one chronic disease like diabetes mellitus, dyslipidemia, hypertension, COPD, thyroid disorders, heart diseases which requires life-long medication. This is further complicated by impairment of special sensory functions like vision and hearing. A decline in immunity as well as age-related physiologic changes leads to an increased burden of communicable diseases or infectious diseases like influenza, pneumonia, tuberculosis (TB) in the elderly population. Most common disabilities among the aged were locomotor and visual, almost half of the elderly disabled population was reported to be suffering from these two types of disabilities (2011 census). Cardiovascular disorders account for one third of elderly mortality followed by respiratory disorders mortality (10%) and infections including TB (10%). It has been reported that a geriatric individual takes an average of six prescription drugs concurrently and often suffers from adverse drug reactions [1, 3, 5, 6].

A key clinical issue in geriatric mental health is the heterogeneity in clinical presentations that confounds diagnosis and treatment of these problems. Patients usually deny the presence of mental health problems and are reluctant to seek help. Geriatric patients have multiple co-morbidities including psychological problems like depression. Few factors contributing to geriatric depression are female sex, widowed status, nuclear families, and stressful life events. Research indicates comparatively higher prevalence of geriatric depression in India, with a median prevalence rate of 21.9%. Symptoms of geriatric depression affect behavioral, physical, and cognitive domains of an individual, while many elderly do not seek help as a stereotype myth prevails that geriatric depression is normal in old age. Dementia is the most common neuropsychiatric illness besides depression as the major contributor to disability in people above 60 years of age, accounting for one quarter of all disability adjusted life years (DALY). It has been shown in different studies that, many environmental factors as well as caregiver approach towards elderly population with dementia are responsible for development of various psychiatric behaviors in elderly like agitation, irritability, restlessness, emotional distress and sleep disturbance. There is urgent need of sufficient number of dementia care homes, rehabilitation centers along with dementia daycare centers to manage the huge number of dementia patients in India [7–12].

2.2 Socioeconomic challenges for the elderly

Elderly or geriatric populations have different socioeconomic problems in their life in the forms of loss of spouse, economic insecurity, social isolation, not getting pension timely etc. Elderly people in India not only work to support themselves but also make economic contributions to their households. Nearly 66% of those over 60 years of age are currently married, 32% are widowed and nearly 3% are separated or divorced (2011 Census). The proportion of those who have lost their spouse is much higher among women compared to men with 48% of older women and only 15% of the older men being widowed. Since women are more likely to be dependent on men for financial security, women face more adversities due to loss of spouse compared to men. Living arrangements among the elderly was not a problem in India till a few years ago because elderly people were given special respect and care in their family. Majority of the elderly are still living with their children in India, about one fifth either live alone or only with the spouse and hence have to manage their material and physical needs on their own. Financial dependency also increases with age. Around 50% of the elderly have some type of personal income after their retirement in the form of social security measures like pension scheme, provident fund, life insurance policies, post office deposits, savings bank interests and non service people of rural as well as urban India get some amount of incentives as part of different national health programs, schemes for elderly population; which will be discussed in subsequent sections. This income earned by the elderly is not sufficient sometimes to fulfill their basic needs and wishes to buy some gifts for their grandchildren on some special occasions. Most of the time, they are seen dependent financially on their offspring. Almost three fourth of the elderly are either fully or partially dependent on others like relatives, friends and neighbors and such dependency is more for elderly women than men. Overall, it appears that elderly still depend greatly on their earnings to support themselves and their family. Presently, lower class and middle class families are facing a great challenge to take care of elderly population due to reduction in economic activities following sudden Covid19 pandemic and subsequent lock-down [1, 6].

3. Covid-19 pandemic situation in India and globally

Corona virus outbreak was first reported in Wuhan city, Hubei province of China at the end of December 2019. Then Italy was affected by this infectious disease followed by multiple countries due to continuous movement of people across the globe by international air travel. The World Health Organization (WHO) declared this Covid outbreak to be a Public Health Emergency of International Concern (PHEIC) on 30th January, 2020. It was declared a pandemic subsequently on 11th March, 2020 when it affected more than hundred (113) countries world-wide [13].

Globally, there have been near about 3 crores (28918900) confirmed cases of COVID-19, with more than 9 lakh (922,252) deaths, reported by WHO with case fatality rate of 3.18% as on, 14 September 2020. Presently, the United States of Americas is at number one position in terms of number of Covid 19 cases, having more than one fifth of total confirmed cases (22.2%) of Covid 19 followed by South-East Asia (18.9%), European region (16.7%), Eastern Mediterranean region (7.3%), African region (3.9%) and Western Pacific (1.9%), being the least affected region globally as on 14th September, 2020. There were more than 1.8 million new cases of COVID-19, with over forty thousand (40,600) deaths reported in the second week of September, 2020.The African Region also showed a decline in Covid 19 cases this week and was the only region to report a decline in deaths due to Covid 19. The European region has reported the third highest number of new cases in this week, accounting for about 16% of global cases and 25% of the deaths, with the second-highest cumulative number of Covid 19 cases per million populations (5,172 cases per million populations). In the South-East Asia Region, three countries namely; India, Indonesia and Bangladesh continue to report the highest number of Covid-19 cases, with the Maldives accounting for the highest number of cumulative cases (16,746 per million populations) in the second week of September, 2020. This region suffered 22% of all new deaths but retains low cumulative deaths in terms of population (46 per million populations). Myanmar is continuing to show increasing number of cases with mortality of less than 1 per million populations. Presently India has the highest number of Covid 19 cases (88.4%) in South-East Asia Region as on 14th September 2020. Indonesia has the highest case fatality rate (4.02%) followed by Thailand (1.67%), India (1.65%), Bangladesh (1.39%), Nepal (0.63%), Myanmar (0.57%), Srilanka (0.37%) and Maldives (0.34%) in South-East Asia Region. Currently, two countries from this region, Bhutan and Timor-Leste have not reported any death due to Covid 19. India has a very good recovery rate of more than 78% till now which is better than many countries compared to huge number of populations affected by Covid 19 [14].

4. Geriatric health care service -need and present scenario in India

Many programmes targeting geriatric population came to act in our country in last few decades but still we do not have the sufficient number of geriatric health clinics, geriatric physicians and caregivers to take care of our elderly. It's high time to look forward in a positive way to deal with these problems of deficiency during this challenging time of Covid 19 pandemic. Geriatrics is relatively a new branch in India with most practicing young physicians having limited knowledge of the clinical and functional implications of aging. India's old, their caregivers and healthcare providers admit ill health as part of senility. Geriatric care is not only concerned with the physiological phenomenon, but also with the medical health problems and specific diseases of an elderly [5].

Increasing elderly population in India together with enhanced awareness on health issues is expected to put considerable pressure on the health care system in general and geriatric care in particular. The United Nations Population Fund (UNFPA) conducted a survey across seven states (Himachal Pradesh, Kerala, Maharashtra, Odisha, Punjab, Tamil Nadu and West Bengal) in India in 2011 to build a knowledge base on the socio-economic and health implications of aging and the ability of the elderly to access and use various welfare initiatives of the government. The survey showed that about 7.6% of the elderly in India (approximately 7.9 million persons) had difficulty in accomplishing activities of daily living (ADLs) and were in need of assistance. In general, elderly women have greater difficulty in performing ADLs than elderly men [1].

Aging of population affects economic development of society as economic productivity is usually carried out by youths and adults - the productive forces. Aging problems vary across different geographical regions depending on demographic diversity, socioeconomic status, cultural and traditional practices. India is a country of demographic heterogeneity and geographical diversity, still one thing is common among its population i.e.; love and respect for each other especially for their elderly population. The family provides social and economic support to individuals at various stages of life. Family transition from joint to nuclear structure affected not only the status of elderly but also the family's capability to care for elderly. Family structure changes were brought out by increased mobility for job opportunity, urbanization, capitalism, division of labor and industrialization. Community based voluntary support and viable formal support systems for elderly with chronic diseases and disabilities might address this issue. Creating provisions for elderly housing, domiciliary care systems, communication technologies might bridge the gap between young and old generations. Demographic factors like very old, women, those living alone and unmarried are more likely to enter long term care institutions. Predictors of social placement of an elderly to an institution are mainly social selection and allocation processes in health delivery systems (theoretical perspective) and risk factors that delay nursing home placement (policy perspective). Important reasons for entry into institutions are unavailability and unwillingness of family members to take care of geriatric population as well as availability of caretaker in private as well as government institution. Conditions viz., living arrangement, perception that institutions are good alternatives and persons involved in decision making in family influence institutionalization of elderly. Institutionalized elderly are heterogeneous in terms of demographic characteristics, physical and mental conditions, service utilization patterns, prognosis and life expectancy. Few factors facilitating entry of elderly people in institution are status of elderly within the family, social issues, existence of nursing home, heterogeneity of nursing homes, behavioral ethnography of nursing home life and resident outcomes and attitude and behavior of nursing home personnel [15].

Over the years, government has launched various schemes with the intention of providing health, care, and independence of the elderly around the country. In the domain of public systems, there are two overarching initiatives that are large in coverage, more comprehensive or integrated in design and backed by financial and administrative resources. These are National programme for Health Care for Elderly (NPHCE) and Integrated Programme for Older Persons (IPOP). They facilitate and create an environment for different kinds of elder services. NPHCE is meant to be implemented in convergence with the National Health Mission, Ministry of AYUSH (Ayurveda, Yoga, Unani, Siddhi and Homeopathy) and the Ministry of Social Justice and Empowerment (MOSJE). The Government of India launched National Policy on Older Persons (NPOP) in 1999 with the primary goal of overall wellbeing of the elderly, ensuring them a legitimate position in the society.

The same Year 1999 was observed as the International year for older persons by the United Nations general assembly. The MOSJE has started the Integrated Programme for Older Persons (IPOP) since 1992, with the aim of improving the quality of life of elderly people by providing basic amenities like food, shelter, medical care and entertainment opportunities. The IPOP provides financial assistance (up to 90%) to Panchayati Raj Institution (PRIs) or local bodies, NGOs, educational institutions, charitable hospitals or nursing homes etc. for initiation of different facilities for elderly like old age homes, mobile medical units for older persons living in rural and isolated areas, day care centers, physiotherapy clinics, provision of disability aids, running help lines and counseling centers and sensitization of school and college students to aging issues [1, 16].

5. National Programme for health Care for Elderly (NPHCE)

Ministry of Health and Family Welfare (MOHFW) is responsible for implementing the National Programme for Health Care of Elderly (NPHCE) through primary, secondary and tertiary services, dedicated for older persons. NPHCE functions under the control, coordination and monitoring and supervision of the national, state and district cells for non-communicable diseases (NCD). NPHCE was launched to provide referral services through district hospitals and regional medical colleges for elderly population and to promote a community based approach for integration of existing primary health centers and capacity building [1, 15, 17].

The Vision of the NPHCE are: (1) Provision of accessible, affordable, and high quality long-term, comprehensive and dedicated care services to elderly population (2) Creation of a new "architecture" for Aging (3) Building a framework for creation of an comfortable environment for "a Society for all Ages;" (4) Promotion of the concept of Active and Healthy Aging.

Specific objectives of the programme are: (1) Provision of an easy access to promotional, preventive, curative and rehabilitative services through community based primary health-care (PHC) approach. (2) Identification of health problems in the elderly and provide appropriate health interventions in the community with a strong referral backup support. (3) Capacity building of the medical and paramedical professionals as well as the caregivers within the family for providing health care to the elderly (4) Provide referral services to the elderly patients through district hospital and regional medical institutions cum colleges.

Few strategies to achieve the above mentioned objectives of the NPHCE are given as mentioned below:

1. Community based PHC approach including domiciliary visits by trained health-care workers (2) Dedicated services at PHC/Community Health Center (CHC) level including provision of machinery, equipment, training, additional human resources, Information, Education and Communication (IEC), etc.

2. Dedicated facilities at the district hospital with 10 bedded wards, additional human resources, machinery and equipment, consumables and drugs, training and IEC

3. Strengthening of Eight Regional Medical Institutes to provide dedicated tertiary level medical facilities for the elderly, introducing PG courses in geriatric medicine, and in-service training of health personnel at all levels

4. Increase use of Information Education Communication (IEC) activities using mass media, folk media and other communication channels to reach out to the vulnerable population

5. Continuous monitoring and independent evaluation of the Program and research in geriatrics and implementation of NPHCE

6. Promotion of public private partnerships in geriatric health-care

7. Mainstreaming AYUSH (Ayurveda, Yoga, Unani, Siddhi and Homeopathy) by revitalization of local health traditions and convergence with programs of Ministry of Social Justice and Empowerment in the field of geriatrics

8. Reorienting traditional medical education to competency based medical education to deal with the problems of geriatric health

Expected outcomes of NPHCE are given as mentioned below:

1. Initiation of Regional geriatric centers (RGC) in eight Regional Medical Institutions by setting up RGCs with a dedicated geriatric out-patient department (OPD) and thirty (30) bedded geriatric ward for management of specific diseases of the elderly, training of health personnel in geriatric health-care and conducting research

2. Generation of Post-graduates in geriatric medicine from the eight regional medical institutions

3. Starting Video Conferencing Units in the eight (8) Regional Medical Institutions to be utilized for capacity building and mentoring

4. Provision of District geriatric units with dedicated geriatric OPD and ten (10) bedded geriatric ward in 80–100 District Hospitals

5. Starting Geriatric clinics or rehabilitation units set up for domiciliary visits in community or primary health centers in the selected districts

6. Strengthening Sub Centers by provision of appropriate logistics like medicines, vaccine carrier etc. and adequate infrastructure like provision for safe drinking water, clean toilet facility, electricity etc.

7. Training of Human Resources in the Public Health-Care System in geriatric care.

8. NPHCE is expected to provide preventive, promotional, curative and rehabilitative services in an integrated manner for the elderly in various Government health facilities. Districts will be linked to Regional Geriatric Centers (RGCs) for providing tertiary level care. Package of services for elderly in different levels of health care delivery system under NPHCE are given in **Table 1**.

5.1 Geriatric health care services in private sector

There are four essential features of an integrated package of elder services in private sector as given below [1]:

1. Affordable medical care at home

2. Improved access to institutional health care while linking home-based care with institution-based services

3. Training staff and family in home-based rehabilitation services

4. Greater participation of the elderly into the society, increasing the level of acceptance by fighting against ageism and continued enjoyment of home life.

While NPHCE and IPOP address aspects related to institutional health care, the rest of the aspects are facilitated by NGOs all over the country with public and private funding. Few NGO initiatives to deal with the health and social problems of elderly in India are as mentioned below:

i. Agewell Foundation

ii. Alzheimer's and Related Disorders Society of India

iii. Calcutta Metropolitan Institute of Gerontology

iv. Ekal Nari Shakti Sangathan (ENSS)

v. Guild for Services

vi. HelpAge India

vii. Heritage Foundation

viii. The International Longevity Centre-India (ILC-I) Elder Care Services

ix. Janaseva Foundation

x. Nightingale Medical Trust

xi. Silver Innings Foundation

xii. Sulabh International services for Widows in Ashrams

6. Conclusion

India is fighting strongly to mitigate the Covid 19 pandemic situation with its limited manpower and economy. Many government programmes and initiatives were launched and coming forward to develop to meet the needs of its vulnerable population like pregnant mother, adolescent, children and elderly since its independence. Public Health Foundation of India has recently launched another programme for training primary health care professionals in Geriatric health care among this most challenging time of Covid 19 pandemic which shows the distant vision of decision makers of health care delivery system in our country. We need to motivate and encourage our young medical graduates to enhance their knowledge and skills in geriatric health to decrease mortality and morbidity in elderly with such types of pandemic in future.

Health facility level	Package of services
Sub-Center (SC)	• Health Education related to healthy ageing
	• Domiciliary visits for attention and care to home bound/bedridden elderly persons and provide training to the family care providers in looking after the disabled elderly persons
	• Arrange for suitable calipers and supportive devices from the PHC to the elderly disabled persons to make them ambulatory
	• Linkage with other support groups and day care centers etc., operational in the area
Primary Health Center (PHC)	• Weekly geriatric clinic run by a trained Medical Officer
	• Maintain a record of the elderly using the standard format during their first visit
	• Conducting a routine health assessment of the elderly persons based on simple clinical examination relating to eye, blood pressure, blood sugar, etc.
	• Provision of medicines and proper advice on chronic ailments
	• Public awareness on promotional, preventive and rehabilitative aspects of geriatrics during health and village sanitation day/camps
	• Referral for diseases needing further investigation and treatment, to CHC or the District Hospital as per need
Community Health Centers (CHC)	• First Referral Unit for the elderly from PHCs and below
	• Geriatric clinic for the elderly persons twice a week
	• Rehabilitation Unit for physiotherapy and counseling
	• Domiciliary visits by the rehabilitation worker for bed ridden elderly and counseling of the family members on their home-based care
	• Health promotion and prevention
	• Referral of difficult cases to District Hospital/higher health-care facility
District hospitals (DH)	• Geriatric clinic for regular dedicated Out Patient Department (OPD) services to the elderly
	• Facilities for laboratory investigations for diagnosis and provision of medicines for geriatric medical and health problems
	• Ten bedded Geriatric Ward for in-patient care of the elderly
	• Existing specialties like General Medicine; Orthopedics, Ophthalmology; ENT services etc., will provide services needed by elderly patients
	• Provide services for the elderly patients referred by the CHCs/PHCs, etc.
	• Conducting camps for Geriatric Services in PHCs/CHCs and other sites
	• Referral services for severe cases to tertiary level hospitals
Regional Geriatric Centers (RGC)	• Geriatric clinic (Specialized OPD for the elderly)
	• Thirty bedded Geriatric Ward for in-patient care and dedicated beds for the elderly patients in the various specialties viz. Surgery, Orthopedics, Psychiatry, Urology, Ophthalmology and Neurology etc.
	• Laboratory investigation required for elderly with a special sample collection center in the OPD block
	• Tertiary health care to the cases referred from medical colleges, district hospitals and below

Table 1.
Package of services for elderly in different levels of health care delivery system under NPHCE are given below.

Acknowledgements

We want to thank **Prof. Partha Bhattacharjee**, Head of department, Community Medicine, Tripura Medical College & Dr. BRAM Teaching Hospital for providing constant encouragement and motivation. Authors want to thank IntechOpen, for giving chance to write in their online platform. Authors also want to express gratitude to Dr. Somchai Amornyotin, Chief Editor, Geriatric book for selecting this chapter on Geriatric Health.

Notes/Thanks/Other declarations

There is no funding agency for this write up. This writing is solely made by the authors with help of different articles and reports. I, **Dr Kaushik Nag** want to thank my wife **Dr Sujata Sen** for constantly motivating and encouraging me for writing this important topic on geriatric health care. I also want to express my gratitude and love towards my parents for guiding me in right direction during my difficult time. I also want to thank my friends cum colleagues for their constant encouragement and motivation. Lastly, I want to express my deepest gratitude and thanks to my geriatric patients without whom this writing would not be possible.

Author details

Kaushik Nag*, Nabarun Karmakar and Anjan Datta
Tripura Medical College and Dr BRAM Teaching Hospital, Agartala, India

*Address all correspondence to: drkaushik86@yahoo.com

References

[1] United Nations Population Fund 2017. 'Caring for Our Elders: Early Responses' - India Ageing Report – 2017. UNFPA, New Delhi, India.

[2] Sundararajan G. Caring for the elderly during the COVID-19 pandemic. UNICEF India. Available at https://www.unicef.org/india/stories/caring-elderly-during-covid-19-pandemic [Accessed: 2020-08-08]

[3] Elderly in India-Profile and Programmes 2016. New Delhi: Ministry of Statistics and Programme Implementation. Government of India. 2016.

[4] World population Aging. 5th report. New York: Population Division of United Nations; 2015. Available at https://www.un.org/en/development/desa/population/publications/pdf/ageing/WPA2015_Report.pdf [Accessed: 2020-08-11]

[5] Khan S and Itrat M. Current Issues in Geriatric Health Care in India-A Review. J Community Med Health Care. 2016; 1(1): 1003.

[6] Census (2011), Primary Census Abstracts, Registrar General of India, Ministry of Home Affairs, Government of India, Available at: http://www.censusindia.gov. in/2011census/PCA/pca_highlights/pe_data.

[7] Lodha P, De Sousa A. Geriatric mental health: The challenges for India. J Geriatr Ment Health 2018;5:16-29.

[8] Jain RK, Aras RY. Depression in geriatric population in urban slums of Mumbai. Indian J Public Health 2007;51:112-3.

[9] Rajkumar AP, Thangadurai P, Senthilkumar P, Gayathri K, Prince M, Jacob KS, et al. Nature, prevalence and factors associated with depression among the elderly in a rural South Indian community. Int Psychogeriatr 2009;21:372-8.

[10] Grover S, Malhotra N. Geriatric depression: A review of Indian research. J Geriatr Ment Health 2015;2:4-15.

[11] Barua A, Ghosh MK, Kar N, Basilio MA. Socio-demographic factors of geriatric depression. Indian J Psychol Med 2010;32:87-92.

[12] Sharma K, Gupta A, Sharma RC, Mahajan N, Mahajan A, Sharma D, et al. Prevalence and risk factors for depression in elderly North Indians. J Geriatr Ment Health 2016;3:158-63.

[13] Khanna RC, Cicinelli MV, Gilbert SS, Honavar SG, Murthy GS. COVID-19 pandemic: Lessons learned and future directions. Indian J Ophthalmol 2020;68:703-10.

[14] Corona Virus Disease (Covid 19): Weekly epidemiological update. available at https://www.who.int/emergencies/diseases/novel-coronavirus-2019/situation-reports/ [Accessed: 2020-09-15]

[15] Salam, Asharaf. (2010). Community based Geriatric care in India: A perspective. Bold: quarterly journal of the International Institute on Aging (United Nations - Malta). 21. 2-16.

[16] Paul NS, Asirvatham M. Geriatric health policy in India: The need for scaling-up implementation. J Family Med Prim Care 2016;5:242-7.

[17] Verma R, Khanna P. National program of health-care for the elderly in India: A hope for healthy ageing. Int J Prev Med 2013;4:1103-7.

Chapter 7

Geriatric Anemia

Manjit Kaur Rana and Amrit Pal Singh Rana

Abstract

Anemia is growing in importance as a public health issue and a biomedical research priority in the geriatric age group but data on the causes and prevalence is not substantial. World health organization (WHO) has defined anemia as hemoglobin concentration (Hb %) below 12 g/dL in women and below 13 g/dL in men. Although it was previously believed that decline in Hb levels might be a normal consequence of aging, later suggested that anemia does reflect underlying poor health and makes elders vulnerable to adverse outcomes. Geriatric anemia has been found to be prevalent in up to 21.1% of patients in Europe and 11.0% of men and 10.2% of women of 65 years and older in the US. There is little literature that explores the various causes of anemia and its association with socio-demographic profile with underlying diseases, hence lesser research has led anemia to go undiagnosed and untreated.

Keywords: geriatric, generalized weakness, unexplained anemia

1. Introduction

Anemia is rising in importance as a biomedical research priority and a public health issue in the old age group. World health organization (WHO) has defined anemia as hemoglobin concentration (Hb %) below 12 g/dL in women and below 13 g/dL in men [1]. Hb declines slightly with more advancing age with frequency of anemia being more pronounced in men. The geriatric anemia is related with mortality and inferior health associated quality of life [2, 3]. This is important area to be explored as there is little literature that explains the association of anemia with old age and lesser research has led anemia to go undiagnosed and untreated. In the shade of absent obvious ailment, complaints of generalized weakness left ignored [4–9]. The incidence of anemia increases comorbidities resulting in increased frequency of hospitalizations hence leading on to adverse impact on survival [10, 11]. So a better outlook is needed to define the optimal Hb levels and to diagnose out the cause of anemia in old age group [12, 13].

2. Definition of anemia and epidemiology

The definition of anemia in the elderly in the literature is controversial. The WHO criteria were established in the 1960s in a cohort lacking individuals >65 years of age [14]. According to WHO criteria anemia was defined as hemoglobin <12 g/dL in women and <13 g/dL in men and absolute iron deficiency was defined as a serum ferritin <30 ng/mL [15, 16]. The National Health and Nutrition Examination Survey

III classifies anemia into four categories as per underlying cause such as anemia from nutritional deficiency, anemia due to renal diseases, anemia of chronic disease and unexplained anemia, in the absence of other specific causes. Worldwide both the number and ratio of older adults growing and there are nearly 500 million (7%) adults, 65 years and older in the world and by 2030 will double to 1 billion (12%). It was predicted that 164 million elderly people who constitute 23.9% of geriatric population were suffering from anemia globally and death risk was elevated to 49% [3, 17]. As per a systematic review the prevalence of anemia was found to be 3–50%. Out of that 3–25% constituted from community-based studies, 31–50% from nursing homes studies and 40–72% hospital admissions [18]. The prevalence of anemia in the institutional studies was observed to be 24%, 31.4%, 46.8%, 54.5%, 66.3%, 67% and 74% in Belgium, Israel, Pakistan, Ethiopia, German, China and US Arespectively [1, 19–23]. Whereas the prevalence of anemia was observed to be 7.3%, 17.7%, 19% and 38% in Turkey, rural India, Iran and urban India respectively in population-based studies [24–27].

3. Clinical features

In elderly, anemia is ignored frequently in spite of obvious evidence that due to decreased Hb levels physiologic functions may worsen in the patients [28]. It has been noticed that there are 75% chances of negligence of symptoms by the patients [29, 30]. Also no related positive finding could be recognized on general physical examinations as there are insufficient signs on physical examination that are specific for mild to moderate anemia [3, 31, 32]. However signs and symptoms vary from weakness, irritability, alopecia, xerostomia and depression especially in iron deficiency anemia (IDA). The restless leg syndrome seen in elderly is also commonly take place with iron deficiency [33–35]. Many studies searched in literature verified that anemia is an independent risk factor for rise in morbidity and mortality along with decreased quality of life in older persons [18, 28, 36–38].

4. Etiopathogenesis

Geriatric anemia to a certain extent may be due to unrevealed underlying diseases or due to reduced bone marrow functional reserve or adaptation to reduced lean body mass with diminished oxygen requirements or escaped erythropoietin secretions. There is plenty of substantiation that hematopoietic stem cells undergo some qualitative changes with age hence resulting in reduced proliferative and regenerative capacity. It has been realized that anemia at older age is rising with the possibly of changes in diagnostics and demographics. Though this also have been emphasized by authors that anemia in the elderly do has a treatable cause [18, 39, 40]. The etiopathogenesis of anemia in geriatric age group is multifaceted and varying from nutritional deficiencies to inflammatory progressions resulting in immunodeficiency. Other causes may be from bone marrow failure syndromes to chronic kidney disease. In general causes of anemia were found to be anemia of chronic disease (ACD) associated with co morbidities, deficiency anemia constituting iron deficiency, vit B 12 deficiency, folate deficiency and others and unexplained anemia. While considering the underlying diseases, anemia in elderly is also seen associated with *H. pylori* and twice prevalent in people with chronic kidney disease (CKD), withprevalence of anemia increasing with stage of CKD [22, 33, 41, 42]. Under normal circumstances, increased plasma and stored iron levels activate Hepcidin production, a hormone released by liver which in turn inhibits dietary iron absorption. Anemia due to iron deficiencies can occur due to low iron content in diet, decreased iron uptake by intestine or excessive bleeding, and compensated by increased erythropoiesis. IDA seemed to be associated with obesity, gastritis and peptic ulcer, esophagitis, Crohn's disease, celiac disease etc. Although, polymedication was considered independent risk factor for anemia, a 12–35% higher chance of anemia was seen in aspirin users alone. Other drugs like corticosteroids and anti-acids were also seen associated with IDA [43, 44]. Screening for under nutrition should be included in assessment of anemia in geriatric patients as low serum albumin levels are found as independent risk factors for anemia in geriatric patients [44, 45]. The association of deficient serum vitamin D levels with anemia is not considered significant as hypoalbuminemia is measured likely to be confounding factor. At the same time as considering the sociodemographic profile as a causative factor, geriatric anemia was significantly seen associated with high socioeconomic status followed by employment and chronic diseases [45, 46]. Another aspect discussed by Freedman ML and associate suggested that low values in elderly especially in men is a physiologic phenomenon or values of anemia need to be revised in this age group is not known [31, 47].

5. Types of anemia

As per National Health and Nutrition Examination Survey III anemia has been classified into four categories as per underlying cause such as anemia from nutritional deficiency, anemia due to renal diseases, anemia of chronic disease and unexplained anemia, in the absence of other specific causes.

Anemia of chronic disease (ACD) is found to be the most common cause of anemia. The prevalence of ACD varies from 33.1–77% in elderly patients (**Table 1**) [1, 37, 48].

The cause of ACD in hospitalized elderly patients is mostly the consequence of added chronic underlying diseases and also is an indicator of several reactive and clonal conditions.3 Many underlying diseases, like H pylori, renal impairment, congestive heart failure, myelodysplastic syndrome (MDS) is seen associated with ACD in elderly [19, 42, 51]. Although concentrations of serum ferritin, white blood counts (WBC) and C-reactive protein (CRP) levels in ACD patients remains high in ACD but high Hepcidin (H) level occurring due to inflammation facilitates development of ACD in elderly patients. Wang WJ et al. have emphasized that best threshold value for the diagnosis of ACD is 130.05 μg/L with the sensitivity of 72% and the specificity of 96% [51–53]. An analysis done by López-Sierra Metal also favored use of serum Transferrin Receptor (sTfR) to check out the state of erythropoiesis in patients with chronic disease [54].

Prevalence	Author's name, year
35%	Joosten E et al., 1992 [1]
65.6%	Chernetsky A et al., 2002 [19]
64%	Willems JM et al., 2012 [49]
77%	Joosten E et al., 2014 [48]
46%	Gowanlock Z et al., 2016 [50]
33.1%	Michalak SS et al., 2018 [37]

Table 1.
Prevalence of anemia of chronic disease in geriatric age group.

Nutritional deficiency anemia is an important clinical problem with prevalence varying from 4% to 22.5% in older patients associated with caloric and protein restriction, iron, vitamin B12, folic deficiency [19, 37, 48, 55]. Protein and energy malnutrition cause an increase in the production of cytokine, stimulation of inflammationand anemia. Due to decreased macrophages activity and ineffective erythropoiesis, reduced red cell mass is seen. In addition, increased cytokines and hepcidin serum levels also seen associated with obesity and underweight [56]. Anemia patients with protein and energy malnutrition more frequently suffered from hypoalbunemia [43]. Absolute IDA is well-defined as anemia with absence of total body iron. To diagnose IDA although serum ferritin is the most often used parameter, but with older age and in the presence of inflammatory diseases concentration of serum ferritin increases and losses its significancy.10Iron deficiency anemia (IDA) contributes approximately 13–15% of total anemia of geriatric age group, mainly associated with underlying diseases.Evidence has been supported by improvement of IDAfrom iron rich diet in geriatric patients [1, 37, 48, 55, 57–59]. New insights into iron homeostasis lead to new diagnostic assays such as serum baseline hepcidin levels could be a useful tool to identify ID in anemic elderly patients. Wang WJ et al. have highlighted thatthe best threshold in diagnosis of IDA was 93.31 μg/L with the sensitivity of 88% and the specificity of 89% [53, 54, 60, 61]. In addition serum transferrin receptor and reticulocyte hemoglobin equivalent is also an emerging investigation to diagnose the disease [54].

Anemia due to CKD fall under the category of decreased RBC production and prevalence varies from 13.2–27% of geriatric anemia [19, 49]. In a smaller number of cases, no clear-cut causes of anemia are identified and when a clear etiopathogenesis is ruled-out the anemia is defined as unexplained anemia (UA) term unexplained anemia. Although the reasons are still under-explored but common pathophysiological mechanisms seems to be associated with an age-related inflammatory process [62, 63]. These patients with unidentified causes are referred to as unexplained anemia or idiopathic cytopenia of unknown significance. The erythropoietin genesis in the kidney becomes suboptimal due to age related affects or changes. This aspect is still underestimated and unexplored while dealing with unexplained anemia. The prevalence of UA varies from 5.8% to 43.7% of the cases (**Table 2**). Many researchers have worked on UA, Price EA and fellows have observed mildly increased inflammatory markers and low erythropoietin levels in patients with this entity. Roy CN and associates have observed that testosterone treatment in case of men 65 years or older with UA and low testosterone levels significantly increased the hemoglobin levels. In testosterone trials, testosterone treatment increased Hb levels in both men who had anemia of a known cause and in men with UA [3, 37, 61, 64–66]. However, similar survival was observed in geriatric patients with UA compared with non-anemic subjects but mortality risks was increased in patients with deficiency anemia compared with non-anemic subjects [49]. The erythropoietin levels seen

Prevalence (%)	Authors name, year
36.8%	Ferrucci L et al., 2007 [64]
43.7%	Artz AS et al. 2011 [23]
35%	Willems JM et al., 2012 [49]
5.8%	Wolff F et al., 2018 [61]
28.4%	Michalak SS, et al., 2018 [37]

Table 2.
Prevalence of unexplained anemia.

inappropriately low in UA indicating that decreased erythropoietin production plays an important role in the pathogenesis of anemia of unknown etiology [50]. On further cytogenetic analysis of UA, one researcher found myelodysplastic syndrome in 4% of the total anemic patients [67]. Whereas in others, present somatic mutations were not found fit as per diagnostic criteria for MDS and condition was termed as clonal cytopenia of undetermined significance [68].

6. Microscopic patterns of anemia

Normocytic anemia being the commonest anemiafollowed by microcytic hypochromic and macrocytic as studied by Kim HS et al. The most common pattern of anemia in a study done by Choi CW has been found to be normocytic anemia amounting to 93.5%, and 3.5% of them being microcytic, and 3% were macrocytic anemias. Bhasin A et al. study showed that most common pattern of anemia as normocytic in 60–90 years age group [69–71].

7. Grade of anemia

WHO classified anemia as public health problem in 2008 into mild, moderate and severe category [72]. Most common grade appreciated is mild (57.1%) with mild to moderate anemia commonly affecting females.While severe and life-threatening anemia is confronted in males predominantly [73]. As greater part of the patients are mild anemia only, foremost findings are difficult to observe even pale conjunctiva usually noted when Hb level drops below 9 gm/dL [32]. So this may be the reason that patients of this grade go unnoticed. For example in a study conducted on 1,146 community-dwelling older females it was found that women with Hb levels of 12 to 13 gm/dL perform worse than women with Hb levels of 13 to 15 gm/dL on tests of walking speed, balance and ability to raise from a chair [74]. Across-sectional study including 334 elderly persons was conducted by Pathiana A and fellows in old age home. The overall prevalence of anemia was found to be 68.7%, 47.4% had mild anemia, 47.0% had moderate anemia and 5.6% had severe anemia with 45% of men with mild anemia as compared to 24.8% in women [30].

It has been suggested in the literature that a diagnostic algorithm should be followed and anemia should be classified with a therapeutic orientation. Supplements of iron, micronutrients and erythropoiesis-stimulating agents should constitute the treatment [75].

8. Conclusion

Anemia in older people is typically mild so it is likely to be overlooked. All elderly persons presenting with health issues should be evaluated for anemia first with complete list of parameters. Proportion and pattern of anemia should be confirmed so that overall outcome and quality of life in case of old age can be improved with specific treatment. Future population-based research is essential for refining for diagnostic testing to tackle out the etiology of geriatric anemia and evaluate effective therapies to reduce the disease burden on the society.

Author details

Manjit Kaur Rana[1*] and Amrit Pal Singh Rana[2]

1 Pathology/Lab Medicine, All India Institute of Medical Sciences, Bathinda, Punjab, India

2 Department of General Surgery, GGS Medical College and Hospital, Faridkot, Punjab, India

*Address all correspondence to: drmrsmanjitkaur@gmail.com

References

[1] Joosten E, Pelemans W, Hiele M, Noyen J, Verhaeghe R, Boogaerts MA. Prevalence and causes of anaemia in a geriatric hospitalized population. Gerontology. 1992;38(1-2):111-117.

[2] Beghé C, Wilson A, Ershler WB. Prevalence and outcomes of anemia in geriatrics: a systematic review of the literature. Am J Med 2004; 116 (Suppl): 3S–10S.

[3] Guralnik JM, Eisenstaedt RS, Ferrucci L, Klein HG, Woodman RC. Prevalence of anemia in persons 65 years and older in the United States: evidence for a high rate of unexplained anemia. Blood 2004; 104: 2263-2268.

[4] De la Cruz-Góngora V, Manrique-Espinoza B, Villalpando S, Téllez-Rojo Solís MM, Salinas-Rodriguez A. Short-term impact of anemia on mortality: evidence from a sample of Mexican older adults. J Aging Health 2014; 26: 750-765.

[5] Hong CH, Falvey C, Harris TB et al. Anemia and risk of dementia in older adults: findings from the Health ABC study. Neurology 2013; 81: 528-533.

[6] Peters R, Burch L, Warner J, Beckett N, Poulter R, Bulpitt C. Haemoglobin, anaemia, dementia and cognitive decline in the elderly, a systematic review. BMC Geriatr 2008;8:18.

[7] Zakai NA, Katz R, Hirsch C et al. A prospective study of anemia status, hemoglobin concentration, and mortality in an elderly cohort. The cardiovascular health study. Arch Intern Med 2005;165:2214-2220.

[8] Izaks G, Westendorp R, Knook D. The definition of anemia in older persons. JAMA 1999;281:3-6.

[9] Joosten E, Lemiengre J, Nels T, Verbeke G, Milisen K. Is anaemia a risk facgtor for delrium in an acute geriatric population? Gerontology. 2006;52:382-385.

[10] Hirani V, Naganathan V, Blyth F et al. Low hemoglobin concentrationa are associatede with sarcopenia, physical performance, and disability in older Australian men in cross-sectional and longitudinal analysis. J GerontolA Biol Sci Med Sci. 2016;71:1667-1675.

[11] Penninx BWJH, Pahor M, Woodman RC, Guralnik JM. Anemia in old age is associated with increased mortality and hospitalization. J GerontolA Biol Sci Med Sci 2006;6474-6479.

[12] . Alexa ID, Ilie AC, Moroşanu A, Voica A. Approaching frailty as the new geriatric syndrome Rev Med Chir Soc Med Nat Iasi. 2013; 117(3):680-685.

[13] Andrès E, Serraj K, Federici L, Vogel T, Kaltenbach G. Anemia in elderly patients: new insight into an old disorder. GeriatrGerontol Int. 2013 Jul;13(3):519-527.

[14] Blanc B, Finch CA, Hallberg L, et al. Nutritional anaemias. Report of a WHO scientific group. World Health Organ Tech Rep Ser. 1968;405:5-37.

[15] World Health Organization. Haemoglobin concentrations for the diagnosis of anaemia and assessment of severity. Geneva, Switzerland: World Health Organization; 2011. [Accessed May 5, 2014]. Available from: http://www.who.int/vmnis/indicators/haemoglobin.pdf.

[16] Ludwig H, Müldür E, Endler G, Hübl W. Prevalence of iron deficiency across different tumors and its association with poor performance status, disease status and anemia. Ann Oncol. 2013;24(7):1886-1892.

[17] United Nations Department of Economic and Social Affairs. Population Division: World Population Prospects. The 2006 Revision. New York: United Nations; 2007.

[18] Gaskell H, Derry S, Moore R, McQuay H. Prevalence of anaemia in older persons: systematic review. BMC Geriatr 2008;8:1-8.

[19] Chernetsky A, Sofer O, Rafael C, Ben-Israel J. Prevalence and etiology of anemia in an institutionalized geriatric population. Harefuah. 2002 Jul;141(7):591-594, 667

[20] Argento V, Roylance J, Skudlarska B, Dainiak N, Amoateng-Adjepong Y. Anemia prevalence in a home visit geriatric population. J Am Med Dir Assoc. 2008;9(6):422-426.

[21] Tariq M, Khalid J, Sania HS, Sarfraz S, Aslam Z, Butt LQ. Morbidity profile of chronic diseases in geriatric patients. J Pak Med Assoc. 2018;68(6):978-981.

[22] Chan TC, Yap DY, Shea YF, Luk JK, Chan FH, Chu LW. Prevalence of anemia in Chinese nursing home older adults: implication of age and renal impairment. Geriatr Gerontol Int. 2013;13(3):591-596.

[23] Artz AS, Fergusson D, Drinka PJ et al. Mechanisms of unexplained anemia in the nursing home. J Am Geriatr Soc 2004; 52: 423-427

[24] Yildirim T, Yalcin A, Atmis V, Cengiz OK, Aras S, Varlı M, Atli T. The prevalence of anemia, iron, vitamin B12, and folic acid deficiencies in community dwelling elderly in Ankara, Turkey. Arch GerontolGeriatr. 2015;60(2):344-348.

[25] Hosseini SR, Zabihi A, Ebrahimi SH, Jafarian Amiri SR, Kheirkhah F, Bijani A. The Prevalence of Anemia and its Association with Depressive Symptoms among Older Adults in North of Iran. J Res Health Sci. 2018;18(4):e00431.

[26] Paul SS, Abraham VJ. How healthy is our geriatric population? a community-based cross-sectional study. J Family Med Prim Care. 2015;4(2):221-225.

[27] Ramachandra SS, Kasthuri A. Anemia in the Elderly Residing in a South Indian Rural Community. Indian Journal for the Practising Doctor. 2008;5(4):2-7.

[28] Penninx BW1, Guralnik JM, Onder G, Ferrucci L, Wallace RB, PahorM.Anemia and decline in physical performance among older persons.Am J Med. 2003;115(2):104-10.

[29] Bach V, Schruckmayer G, Sam I et al. Prevalence and possible causes of anemia in the elderly: a cross-sectional analysis of a large European university hospital cohort. Clin Interv Aging. 2014;9:1187-1196.

[30] Pathania A, Haldar P, Kant S, Gupta SK, Pandav CS, Bachani D. Prevalence of anaemia among elderly persons residing in old age homes in national capital territory, Delhi, India. Indian J Public Health 2019;63:288-292.

[31] Sanford AM, Morley JE. Anemia of Old Age. J Nutr Health Aging. 2019;23:602-605.

[32] Kalantri A, Karambelkar M, Joshi R et al. Accuracy and reliability of pallor for detecting anaemia: A hospital-based diagnostic accuracy study. PLoS One. 2010;5(1):e8545.

[33] Vetrano DL, Zucchelli A, Marconi E, Levi M, Pegoraro V, Cataldo N, Heiman F, Cricelli C, Lapi F. Predictors of iron-deficiency anemia in primary care older adults: a real-world European multi-country

longitudinal study. Aging Clin Exp Res. 2020;32(11):2211-2216.

[34] Lieske B, Röhrig G, Becker I, Schulz RJ, Polidori MC, Kassubek J. StationärbehandeltegeriatrischePatientenmitEisenmangel-assoziiertem Restless-Legs-Syndrom : Eine retrospektiveAnalyse [Geriatric inpatients with iron deficiency-associated Restless Legs Syndrome. A retrospective analysis]. MMW Fortschr Med. 2017;159(4):12-17.

[35] Stewart, Robert MD; Hirani, Vasant MSc Relationship Between Depressive Symptoms, Anemia, and Iron Status in Older Residents From a National Survey Population, Psychosomatic Medicine: February/March 2012;74(2):208-213

[36] Gandhi SJ, Hagans I, Nathan K ET AL. Prevalence, Comorbidity and Investigation of Anemia in the Primary Care Office. J Clin Med Res. 2017;9(12):970-980.

[37] Michalak S, Rupa-Matysek J, Gil L. Comorbidities, repeated hospitalizations, and age ≥ 80 yearsas indicators of anemia development in the older population. Ann Hematol. 2018;97:1337-1347.

[38] Den Elzen WPJ, Willems JM, Westendorp RGJ, De CraenAJM, Assendelft WJJ, Gussekloo J. Effect of anaemia and comorbidity on functional status and mortality in old age: results from the Leiden 85-plus Study. CMAJ. 2009;181(3-4):151-157.

[39] Price EA. Aging and erythropoiesis: Current state of knowledge. Blood Cells, Molecules, and Diseases. 2008;41:158-165.

[40] Beerman I, Seita J, Inlay MA et al. Quiescent Hematopoietic Stem Cells Accumulate DNA Damage during Aging that Is Repaired upon Entry into Cell Cycle. Cell Stem Cell. 2014;15:37-50.

[41] Stauffer ME, Fan T. Prevalence of anemia in chronic kidney disease in the United States. PLoS One. 2014;9(1):e84943.

[42] Hou B, Zhang M, Liu M, Dai W, Lin Y, Li Y, Gong M, Wang G. Association of active Helicobacter pylori infection and anemia in elderly males. BMC Infect Dis. 2019;19(1):228.

[43] Röhrig G, Rücker Y, Becker I, Schulz RJ, Lenzen-Großimlinghaus R, Willschrei P, Gebauer S, Modreker M, Jäger M, Wirth R. Association of anemia with functional and nutritional status in the German multicenter study "GeriAnaemie2013". Z GerontolGeriatr. 2017 Aug;50(6):532-537.

[44] Frangos E, Trombetti A, Graf CE, Lachat V, Samaras N, Vischer UM, Zekry D, Rizzoli R, Herrmann FR. Malnutrition in Very Old Hospitalized Patients: A New Etiologic Factor of Anemia? J Nutr Health Aging. 2016;20(7):705-713.

[45] Coutard A, Garlantézec R, Estivin S, Andro M, Gentric A. Association of vitamin D deficiency and anemia in a hospitalized geriatric population: denutrition as a confounding factor. Ann Hematol. 2013 May;92(5):615-619.

[46] Ernst JB, Prokop S, Fuchs U, Dreier J, Kuhn J, Knabbe C, Berthold HK, Pilz S, Gouni-Berthold I, Gummert JF, Börgermann J, Zittermann A. Randomized supplementation of 4000 IU vitamin D3 daily vs placebo on the prevalence of anemia in advanced heart failure: the EVITA trial. Nutr J. 2017;16(1):49.

[47] Freedman ML, Marcus DL. Anemia and the elderly: is it physiology or pathology? Am J Med Sci. 1980;280:81-85.

[48] Joosten E, Lioen P. Iron deficiency anemia and anemia of chronic disease in geriatric hospitalized patients:

How frequent are comorbidities as an additional explanation for the anemia? Geriatr Gerontol Int 2015;15: 931-935.

[49] Willems JM, den Elzen WP, Vlasveld LT, Westendorp RG, Gussekloo J, de Craen AJ, Blauw GJ. No increased mortality risk in older persons with unexplained anaemia. Age Ageing. 2012;41(4):501-506.

[50] Gowanlock Z, Sriram S, Martin A, Xenocostas A, Lazo-Langner A. Erythropoietin Levels in Elderly Patients with Anemia of Unknown Etiology. PLoS One. 2016 Jun 16;11(6):e0157279.

[51] Solomakhina NI, Nakhodnova ES, Belenkov YN. [Anemia of chronic disease and iron deficiency anemia: Comparative characteristics of ferrokinetic parameters and their relationship with inflammation in late middle-aged and elderly patients with CHF]. Kardiologiia. 2018 SAug;58(Suppl 8):58-64.

[52] Stauder R, Valent P, Theurl I. Anemia at older age: etiologies, clinical implications, and management. Blood. 2018 Feb 1;131(5):505-514.

[53] Wang WJ, Wang H, Chen Z, Chen Y. [Diagnostic value of hepcidin in elderly patients with iron deficiency anemia and anemia of chronic disease]. Zhongguo Shi Yan Xue Ye Xue Za Zhi. 2015 Feb;23(1):155-8. Chinese. doi: 10.7534/j.issn.1009-2137.2015.01.030. PMID: 25687065.

[54] López-Sierra M, Calderón S, Gómez J, Pilleux L. Prevalence of Anaemia and Evaluation of Transferrin Receptor (sTfR) in the Diagnosis of Iron Deficiency in the Hospitalized Elderly Patients: Anaemia Clinical Studies in Chile. Anemia. 2012;2012:646201.

[55] Sturtzel B, Elmadfa I, Hermann B, Schippinger W, Ohrenberger G. Effects of an enhanced iron dense foods offering in the daily meals served in geriatric institutions on measures of iron deficiency anemia. BMC Geriatr. 2018;18(1):123.

[56] Bianchi VE. Role of nutrition on anemia in elderly. Clin Nutr ESPEN. 2016 Feb;11:e1-e11.

[57] Gómez M, Ble M, Cladellas M, Molina L, Comín-Colet J, Enjuanes C, Roqueta C, Soler C, Bruguera J. Effect of correction of anemia on echocardiographic and clinical parameters in patients with aortic stenosis involving a three-cuspid aortic valve and normal left ventricular ejection fraction. Am J Cardiol. 2015 Jul 15;116(2):270-274.

[58] Helsen T, Joosten E. IJzergebreksanemiebijouderen [Iron deficiency in the elderly]. TijdschrGerontolGeriatr. 2016 Jun;47(3):109-116.

[59] Joosten E. Iron deficiency anemia in older adults: A review. GeriatrGerontol Int. 2018 Mar;18(3):373-379.

[60] Epub 2015 Apr 18. PMID: 25983280. 7Auerbach M, Spivak J. Treatment of Iron Deficiency in the Elderly: A New Paradigm. Clin Geriatr Med. 2019;35(3):307-317.

[61] Wolff F, De Breucker S, Pepersack T, Compté N, Mélot C, Gulbis B, Cotton F. Baseline hepcidin measurement in the differential diagnosis of anaemia for elderly patients and its correlation with the increment of transferrin saturation following an oral iron absorption test. Clin Chem Lab Med. 2018;57(2):250-258.

[62] Halawi R, Moukhadder H, Taher A. Anemia in the elderly: a consequence of aging? Expert Rev Hematol. 2017 Apr;10(4):327-335.

[63] Cappellini MD, Motta I. Anemia in Clinical Practice-Definition and Classification: Does Hemoglobin

Change With Aging? Semin Hematol. 2015 Oct;52(4):261-269.

[64] Ferrucci L, Guralnik JM, Bandinelli S, Semba RD, Lauretani F, Corsi A, Ruggiero C, Ershler WB, Longo DL. Unexplained anaemia in older persons is characterised by low erythropoietin and low levels of pro-inflammatory markers. Br J Haematol. 2007;136(6):849-855.

[65] Roy CN, Snyder PJ, Stephens-Shields AJ, et al. Association of Testosterone Levels With Anemia in Older Men: A Controlled Clinical Trial [published correction appears in JAMA Intern Med. 2019 Mar 1;179(3):457]. JAMA Intern Med. 2017;177(4):480-490.

[66] Snyder PJ, Bhasin S, Cunningham GR, Matsumoto AM, Stephens-Shields AJ et al. Lessons From the Testosterone Trials. Endocr Rev. 2018;39(3):369-386.

[67] Pang WW, Schrier SL. Anemia in the elderly. CurrOpinHematol. 2012;19(3):133-140.

[68] Stauder R, Valent P, Theurl I. Anemia at older age: etiologies, clinical implications, and management. Blood. 2018 Feb 1;131(5):505-514.

[69] Choi CW, Lee J, Park KH et al. Prevalence and characteristics of anemia in the elderly: Cross-sectional study of three urban Korean population samples. American Journal of Hematology. 2004;77:26-30.

[70] Kim HS, Lee BK. Cross-sectional study on the prevalence of anemia among rural elderly in Asan. Nutr Res Pract. 2008;2(1):8-12.

[71] Bhasin A, Medha R. Characteristics of Anemia in Elderly: A Hospital Based Study in South India. Indian journal of hematology & blood transfusion: an official journal of Indian Society of Hematology and Blood Transfusion. 2011;27:26-32.

[72] Benoist BD, Erin ML, Ines E et al. Worldwide prevalence of anemia. 1993-2005: WHO global database on anemia. Spain: WHO.2008.

[73] ErshlerWB, ShengSH, McKelvey Jet al. Serum Erythropoietin and Aging: A Longitudinal Analysis. 2005;53(8):1360-1365.

[74] Chaves PHM, XueQL,Guralnik JM et al. What Constitutes Normal Hemoglobin Concentration in Community-Dwelling Disabled Older Women?2004;52:1811-6.

[75] Gómez Ramírez S, Remacha Sevilla ÁF, Muñoz Gómez M. Anaemia in the elderly. Med Clin (Barc). 2017;149(11):496-503.

Chapter 8

Assessing Anticholinergic Effects in Older Adults

Donna M. Lisi

Abstract

Anticholinergic medications are widely used in older adults and are a common source of adverse events in this population. Common drug classes include antiarrhythmics, antidepressants, antiemetics, first generation antihistamines, urinary incontinence antimuscarinic agents, antiparkinsonian agents, antipsychotics, antispasmodics, and skeletal muscle relaxants. These drugs have been associated with delirium, cognitive impairment, sedation, dizziness, falls, fracture, constipation, urinary retention, blurred vision, tachycardia and dry mouth. If possible, these drugs should be avoided in older adults or less toxic agents within the class should be utilized. This chapter will explore the mechanism of action of anticholinergic drugs at both the cellular and organ system level; discuss how to assess for anticholinergic drug burden; list medications with anticholinergic effects as identified in the Beer's criteria on potentially inappropriate medication use in older adults; review anticholinergic drug–drug interactions; describe contraindications to the use of anticholinergic agents; and explore practical considerations such as the availability of these substances in nonprescription medications, their use at end of life and deprescribing.

Keywords: anticholinergic medications, Beer's criteria, adverse drug events, older adults, geriatrics

1. Introduction

1.1 Anticholinergic agents in nature

Anticholinergic agents are substances that antagonize the effects of acetylcholine, a neurotransmitter formed by an ester of choline and acetic acid, that facilitates nerve impulses in both the central (CNS) and peripheral nervous systems. Acetylcholine is the main neurotransmitter of the parasympathetic system. It is also located within parts of the autonomic nervous system [1]. Anticholinergic agents are present in both pharmaceuticals and in nature. Substances like hyoscyamine and belladonna are naturally occurring anticholinergics which have been used medicinally to control gastric secretions, for irritable bowel symptoms, and for urinary spasms [2]. However, despite their natural origins, the use of these drugs is not without consequence and should be avoided in older adults.

2. Anticholinergics physiological effects

2.1 Mechanisms of action

The cholinergic receptors are divided into muscarinic receptors or nicotinic receptors. There are five subtypes of muscarinic receptors, M1-M5 and two types of nicotinic receptors, N_M (skeletal muscle) and N_N (neuronal). M1 are found in the CNS (i.e., the cerebral cortex, hippocampus, striatum and thalamus), autonomic ganglia, gastric and salivary glands and the enteric nerves of the GI tract. M2 are located in the CNS (i.e., the hindbrain, thalamus, cerebral cortex, hippocampus, striatum, heart, smooth muscle, and autonomic nerve terminals). M3 receptors have less of a presence in the CNS although they are found in the cerebral cortex and hippocampus. They are abundant in smooth muscle and glands and the heart. M4 is preferentially expressed in the CNS (i.e., forebrain, striatum, cerebral cortex and hippocampus) while M5 are only expressed in low levels in the CNS and periphery and are found primarily in the substantia nigra and ventral tegmentum area. N_M are located at the neuromuscular junction and are involved in muscle contraction. Nn are found in the autonomic ganglia and adrenal medulla [3].

At the cellular level, anticholinergic agents act by opposing the effects of acetylcholine either at the muscarinic or nicotinic receptors. In the geriatric population, most anticholinergic drugs affect the muscarinic receptors. On the organ system level, these compounds have varying effects. Although some effects are therapeutic, it's their toxic effects that are most worrisome, especially in geriatric patients.

While M1-M5 receptors are found in the brain, most of the deleterious effects on the CNS come from antagonizing M1 receptors. This can lead to delirium, cognitive impairment, dizziness, sedation and confusion. The predominant form of muscarinic receptors in the eyes are M3 although M1-M5 receptors are also present. Blocking these receptors leads to mydriasis and blurred vision. It is for this reason that ophthalmic atropine, a potent anticholinergic agent, is used to produce pupillary dilation and/or cycloplegia. Blocking of M1 and M3 receptors in salivary glands leads to dry mouth and difficulty swallowing whereas opposing the effects of M3 receptors in sweat glands leads to the inability to dissipate heat and can result in overheating, especially during the warmer months. The heart is primarily composed of M2 receptors and antagonizing these receptors leads to sinus tachycardia and increased contractility. Systemic atropine is used in the management of symptomatic sinus bradycardia and atrioventricular nodal block. The lungs primarily contain M1-M4 receptors and blocking these receptors results in bronchodilation. The use of long- and short-acting inhalation antimuscarinic agents in chronic obstructive pulmonary disease (COPD) takes advantage of this beneficial effect. Opposing M2 and M3 receptors in the GI tract can lead to gastric stasis and constipation. On the other hand, dicyclomine is an anticholinergic drug that is used for abdominal pain associated with irritable bowel syndrome. Antagonism of M3 receptors in the bladder inhibits detrusor and bladder contractions and is used therapeutically for urinary incontinence. This blockade can also lead to urinary retention. The role of cholinergic agents in the skin, which contains primarily M3 receptors, is complex resulting in increased nitric oxide production and vasodilation and it also involves interplay with nicotinic receptors [4].

Nicotinic agents act either as neuromuscular blockers (i.e., atracurium, vecuronium, tubocurarine, pancuronium) or ganglionic blockers (i.e., mecamylamine). Succinylcholine is a N_M receptor agonist [4].

3. Assessment of anticholinergic burden

The effects of anticholinergic agents are cumulative and there are various tools available to help evaluate the degree of 'cholinergic burden' in an older adult's drug regimen. Early work by Tune et al. resulted in the development of the serum anticholinergic assay, a biologic measure intended to quantify anticholinergic drug burden [5]. Using this assay, it has been shown that many drugs taken by older adults have high serum anticholinergic activity **Table 1** [6].

Over 600 medications have some degree of anticholinergic activity [7]. One drawback of using the serum anticholinergic assay is that it may not be readily available in clinical settings and even if available, there can be a delay in care pending interpretation of results [8].

As a result of these limitations, scales have been developed to easily calculate the cumulative anticholinergic burden. The Anticholinergic Cognitive Burden Scale (ACBS) rates drugs on a scale of 0 (no anticholinergic effect) to 3 with 1 representing a possible anticholinergic effect based on laboratory tests but no evidence of clinically relevant cognitive effects and scores of 2 or 3 indicating definite anticholinergic effects. Higher scores indicate greater anticholinergic burden and warrant a re-evaluation of the drug regimen. The presence of a drug scoring 2 or 3 can increase the risk of cognitive impairment by 46% over 6 years. Further, each point increase in the ACBS has been associated with a decrease in the Mini-Mental Examination Score of 0.33 points over the course of 2 years. This point increase has also been associated with a 26% increase in the risk of death [9].

Another tool is the Anticholinergic Risk Scale (ARS). Similar to ACBS, the ARS is also a 3-point scale. The developers of the scale assessed whether the ARS could predict the risk of anticholinergic adverse effects in a geriatric evaluation and management (GEM) group and in a primary care (PC) group. The investigators found that in the GEM group, older adults experienced more adverse CNS effects whereas in the PC group, more elderly had peripheral adverse effects [10].

The Anticholinergic Drug Scale (ADS), which was previously known as the Clinician-Rated Anticholinergic Scale, is another 3-point scale. It includes the

Medications	Anticholinergic Drug Level (ng/mL Atropine)
Cimetidine	0.86
Prednisolone	0.55
Theophylline	0.44
Digoxin	0.25
Furosemide	0.22
Nifedipine	0.22
Ranitidine	0.22
Isosorbide dinitrate	0.15
Warfarin	0.12
Codeine	0.11
Triamterene/HCTZ	0.08
Captopril	0.02

Table 1.
Anticholinergic drug level of medications commonly used by older adults.

largest number of anticholinergic agents. A score of 0 indicates no known anticholinergic properties; a score of 1 means that the drug has the potential for anticholinergic activity as evidenced by receptor binding sites; a score of 2 represents a drug that causes anticholinergic adverse effects at higher doses; and a score of 3 represents a drug with marked anticholinergic activity [11].

The Anticholinergic Burden Classification (ABC) measures serum anticholinergic activity but takes into account the duration of exposure, adjusts for mode of administration (i.e., topical, nasal, oral, etc.), assesses for possible drug–drug interactions and for the ability of drugs to cross the blood brain barrier [12].

The Anticholinergic Activity Scale (AAS) is based on *in vivo* radioreceptor assay determinations and ranks drugs on five levels: 0 (no anticholinergic activity); 0/+ (no or minimal anticholinergic activity); + (low anticholinergic activity), ++ (moderate anticholinergic activity), and +++ (high anticholinergic activity) [13].

The Anticholinergic Loading Scale (ALS) is a tool used in the Australian Imaging, Biomarkers and Lifestyle (AIBL) study that calculates anticholinergic load. Anticholinergic load was found to have an adverse effect on psychomotor speed and executive function in healthy controls [14].

The Anticholinergic Effect on Cognition Scale (AECS) is another 3-point scale that uses *in vitro* anticholinergic potency as well as a drug's ability to cross the blood brain barrier [15].

Unlike the previous scales, which only focus on the anticholinergic potential of a drug regimen, the Drug Burden Index (DBI) takes into account anticholinergic effects, sedative effects of medications, and the total number of medications. It measures the effect of cumulative exposure to both anticholinergic and sedative medications on physical and cognitive function in older adults. This scale is based on the *minimum recommended daily doses* of each drug. Drugs that have both anticholinergic and sedative properties are classified based on their anticholinergic effects [16]. The developers studied this scale in over 3000 healthy community-dwelling older adults aged 70–79 years. They found that the use of anticholinergic and sedative medications was associated with poorer physical performance and cognitive performance. Each unit of drug burden on physical function was equal to having three additional physical comorbidities whereas each unit of drug burden on cognition was similar to having four additional physical comorbidities or about half of the effects of anxiety, depression or cognitive impairment [17].

A recent publication compared several of the anticholinergic scales providing a description of the tool and listing the number of drugs with anticholinergic activity that are included in the scale [18]. However, while many of these scales have shown a significant correlation between anticholinergic burden assessment and serum anticholinergic drug levels, they have limitations. There is currently no 'gold standard' to identify an *anticholinergic drug*. Only parent compounds are included in these scales, therefore, there is no information on active metabolites that may also contribute to the anticholinergic burden. While some scales do take dose into the account, this is not consistently done in all tools. These scales also assume that there is a linear relationship between anticholinergic levels and toxicity. Lastly, serum anticholinergic activity assays do not distinguish between agonist versus antagonist binding of the cholinergic receptors [19].

4. Medication classes with anticholinergic effects- the Beer's list of potentially inappropriate medications in older adults

In 1991, Dr. Mark Beers published explicit criteria for the use of 'potentially inappropriate medications' or PIMS in older nursing home residents [20]. The

Drug Class	Specific Drugs
Antiarrhythmics	Disopyramide
Antidepressants	Amitriptyline, amoxapine, clomipramine, desipramine, doxepin (> 6 mg), imipramine, nortriptyline, paroxetine, protriptyline, trimipramine
Antiemetics	Prochlorperazine, promethazine
First Generation Antihistamines	Brompheniramine, carbinoxamine, chlorpheniramine, clemastine, cyproheptadine, dexbrompheniramine, dexchlorpheniramine, dimenhydrinate, diphenhydramine (oral), doxylamine, hydroxyzine, meclizine, clidinium-chlordiazepoxide, dicyclomine, homatropine (except ophthalmic), hyoscyamine, methscopolamine, propantheline, promethazine, pyrilamine, triprolidine
Urinary Incontinence Antimuscarinics	Darifenacin, fesoterodine, flavoxate, oxybutynin, solifenacin, tolterodine, trospium
Antiparkinsonian Agents	Benztropine, trihexyphenidyl
Antipsychotics	Chlorpromazine, clozapine, loxapine, olanzapine, perphenazine, thioridazine, trifluoperazine
Antispasmodics	Atropine (except ophthalmic), belladonna alkaloids, scopolamine (except ophthalmic)
Skeletal Muscle Relaxants	Cyclobenzaprine, orphenadrine

Table 2.
Beer's list drugs with strong anticholinergic properties.

Beer's criteria, which were developed using a two-stage Delphi survey, defined inappropriate prescribing as the use of a medication where the potential risks outweigh the potential benefits. These initial criteria included 30 therapeutic classes/medications that should be avoided in elderly nursing home residents [21]. This list is updated every 3 years by the American Geriatrics Society. At the time of this writing, the latest Beer's List was published in 2019. The criteria identifies PIMs, drugs that may be PIMS because they may exacerbate disease states or geriatric syndromes, drugs that should be used with caution, drugs that should be avoided, drugs that should be used in reduced doses (if at all) based on renal function, and drugs with strong anticholinergic properties **Table 2** [22].

5. Adverse effects of anticholinergics ("Alice in Wonderland")

As mentioned previously, cholinergic receptors are found in various organ systems throughout the body. Blocking these receptors can have both therapeutic and toxic effects. The mnemonic "red as a beet, dry as a bone, blind as a bat, mad as a hatter, hot as a hare, full as a flask" reflects the classic signs and symptoms of anticholinergic poisoning [23]. However, adverse events in older adults may be more subtle. These can include drowsiness, sedation, cognitive impairment, confusion, delirium, hallucinations, blurred vision, dizziness, falls/fractures, urinary retention, constipation, tachycardia, and xerostomia [3, 22].

Adverse CNS effects can be particularly burdensome among older adults. A recent study examining the effects of PIMs in patients with dementia found that almost one-quarter of adults aged ≥65 with cognitive impairment used drugs with clinically significant anticholinergic effects. This study measured anticholinergic burden using the ADS [11]. It found that the level 2 drugs that were most prescribed were ranitidine and cyclobenzaprine and the most commonly prescribed level 3 drugs were meclizine, tolterodine and oxybutynin [24]. A systematic review examining drug-induced delirium found that ARS scores were consistently associated with delirium [25]. A recent retrospective analysis found that if older hospitalized adults scored 3 or higher on the ACBS, they had a 3–6 fold increased risk of developing delirium compared to those who score < 3 on this tool [26]. In older adults with mild to moderate Alzheimer's disease who were APOE-ε4 carriers, there was a positive correlation between greater progression of dementia severity and continued use of anticholinergic medications [27].

In addition to the CNS effects of anticholinergic agents in older adults, another concern is the risk of falls and fracture. After following women with a mean age of 55 years for approximately 24 months, the APOS (Aberdeen Prospective Osteoporosis Screening Study) found that those with a ACB of ≥2 had a 2.34-fold increased odds of having had recurrent falls in 'later life' with 'later life' referring to 12 months prior to follow-up; there was a 2-year follow-up period. They postulated that anticholinergic agents may contribute to falls by causing vision problems secondary to pupillary dilation, dizziness, slowed reflexes and/or cognitive impairment [28].

Death, the most significant anticholinergic adverse event, was observed in a systematic review of studies examining the association between anticholinergic burden and mortality in older adults. Of the 27 studies included in this systematic review, 63% of studies found a positive relationship between anticholinergic drug burden and mortality in older adults. When solely analyzing those studies that were deemed to be of the *highest quality*, the association between anticholinergic drug use and death rose to 80% in the elderly [29].

6. Drug interactions involving anticholinergic agents

Besides the anticholinergic drug–drug interactions that lead to an increased anticholinergic burden, anticholinergic agents are involved in other potential drug–drug interactions.

The use of an anticholinergic agent with an acetylcholinesterase inhibitor (i.e., donepezil, galantamine and rivastigmine) results in opposing pharmacodynamic effects and can negate any small, positive benefits seen with the Alzheimer's disease agents [30]. Conversely, acetylcholinesterase inhibitors have the potential to interfere with the therapeutic effects of anticholinergic agents. Concomitant use is not recommended [31–33].

The concomitant administration of an anticholinergic agent and an oral solid dosage form of potassium supplement can increase the risk of GI bleeding. A liquid formulation of potassium supplement should be utilized instead if concurrent therapy is required [34–36].

Anticholinergic agents also interact with carbonic anhydrase inhibitors such as topiramate and zonisamide potentiating the risk of oligohidrosis and hyperthermia. Patients should be monitored for decreased sweating and increases in body temperature. These combinations should be avoided [37, 38].

Concurrent use of opioids and anticholinergics can lead to severe constipation (resulting in paralytic ileus), sedation, dizziness, confusion, cognitive and psychomotor impairment, dry mouth and urinary retention. Caution is advised [39].

'Moderate' (i.e., drug–drug interactions for which combination therapy should be avoided or used only under special circumstances) anticholinergic drug–drug interactions include abobotulinumtoxin A, acebutolol, acetylcholine ophthalmic, aclidinium, acrivastine, alfentanil, aluminum hydroxide, amantadine, ambenonium, amitriptyline, amoxapine, arbutamine, aripiprazole, asenapine, atenolol, azatadine, belladonna, benztropine, betaxolol, bethanechol, biperiden, bisoprolol, brexanolone, brexpiprazole, brompheniramine, buprenorphine, butorphanol, calcium carbonate, carbachol ophthalmic, carbinoxamine, cariprazine, carteolol, carvedilol, cevimeline, chlorcyclizine, chlorpheniramine, chlorpromazine, cisapride, clemastine, clidinium, clomipramine, clozapine, cyclizine, cyclobenzaprine, cyproheptadine, darifenacin, demecarium bromide ophthalmic, desipramine, dexbrompheniramine, dexchlorpheniramine, dezocine, dicyclomine, dimenhydrinate, diphenhydramine, disopyramide, doxepin, doxylamine, echothiophate iodide ophthalmic, edrophonium, eluxadoline, ethanol, fesoterodine, flavoxate, flibanserin, fluphenazine, glycopyrrolate, glycopyrronium topical, guanidine, haloperidol, hydroxyzine, hyoscyamine, iloperidone, imipramine, incobotulinumtoxin A, ipratropium, isoflurophate ophathalmic, kaolin, ketoconazole, labetalol, lasmiditan, levodopa, loperamide, loxapine, lumateperone, lurasidone, macimorelin, magaldrate, magnesium carbonate, magnesium hydroxide, maprotiline, meclizine, memantine, mepenzolate, mesoridazine, methdilazine, methotrimeprazine, methscopolamine, metoclopramide, metoprolol, molindone, nadolol, nalbuphine, nebivolol, neostigmine, nortriptyline, olanzapine, olopatadine nasal, onabotulinumtoxin A, orphenadrine, oxybutynin, paliperidone, penbutolol, perphenazine, phenindamine, phenylephrine, physostigmine, pilocarpine, pimozide, pindolol, prabotulinumtoxin A, pramlintide, prochlorperazine, procyclidine, promazine, promethazine, propantheline, propiomazine, propranolol, protriptyline, prucalopride, pyridostigmine, pyrilamine, quetiapine, quinapril, remifentanil, revefenacin, rimabotulinumtoxin B, risperidone, scopolamine, sodium bicarbonate, solifenacin, sotalol, sufentanil, thiethylperazine, thioridazine, thiothixene, timolol, tiotropium, tizanidine, tolterodine, trifluoperazine, triflupromazine, trihexyphenidyl, trimeprazine, trimipramine, tripelennamine, triprolidine, trospium, umeclidinium and ziprasidone [40].

7. Contraindications to the use of anticholinergic agents

Anticholinergic agents cause pupillary dilation, which is detrimental in patients with narrow angle or primary angle closure glaucoma. When the pupils dilate, this increases pressure within the eye. This increase in pressure prevents drainage of aqueous humor from the eye resulting in marked increases in ocular pressure and acute pain. If left untreated, this can lead to optic nerve damage and vision loss. The use of anticholinergics is contraindicated in patients with this type of glaucoma [41].

In overactive bladder, there are excessive contractions of the detrusor muscle producing incomplete emptying of the bladder. By blocking M3 receptors in the genitourinary tract, this causes smooth muscle relaxation and detrusor underactivity, which can lead to urinary retention. In the presence of benign prostate hyperplasia, there is compression of the urethra, which blocks the flow of urine. Anticholinergic agents are contraindicated in patients with urinary retention and bladder neck obstruction caused by prostatic hypertrophy since the use of these agents can result in an increased risk of developing an obstructive uropathy [42].

Myasthenia gravis is an autoimmune disorder of the postsynaptic neuromuscular junction caused by antibody-mediated blockade of neuromuscular transmission that results in skeletal muscle weakness. Autoimmune antibodies form at the neuromuscular junction against nicotinic acetylcholine postsynaptic receptors. Anticholinergics, especially agents that block nicotinic cholinergic receptors, are contraindicated because they exacerbate muscle weakness. Further, acetylcholine esterase inhibitors such as pyridostigmine are considered the mainstay of treatment. The use of anticholinergic agents would antagonize the effects of these drugs [42, 43].

Stimulation of M1 and M2 receptors in the GI tract increases GI motility. Anticholinergics block these receptors resulting in slowed GI motility. Ogilive's syndrome or colonic pseudo-obstruction, which is massive dilation of the colon without underlying mechanical obstruction or other organic causes, can be due to the use of anticholinergic agents. These drugs can lead to an adynamic colon. Anticholinergic drugs are contraindicated in patients with achalasia, esophageal stricture or stenosis, pyloroduodenal stenosing peptic ulcer disease, pyloric obstruction and paralytic ileus [42, 44].

Stimulation of M2 receptors in the heart slow pacemaker activity and atrioventricular (AV) conduction, which decreases contractility. Blocking these receptors leads to sinus tachycardia and increased oxygen demand [45]. Analyses of data from the EPIC (European Prospective Investigation into Cancer)-Norfolk Population Study, which was a longitudinal, observation, community cohort study, found that among the 21,000 study participants there was an increase in total anticholinergic burden and subsequent risk of all-cause mortality and incident cardiovascular disease during the follow up period. ACBS scores of ≥3 were associated with a hazard ratio of 2.17 ($p < 0.00001$) for cardiovascular disease incidence and higher mortality. It was thought that this was a dose-dependent, class effect for the anticholinergic agents. Potential mechanisms of this effect could be a pro-arrhythmic or pro-ischemic effect, increased hemodynamic lability, cardiac ischemia, cardiac dysrhythmias in the presence of ischemia, decrease heart rate variability, or an inflammatory response resulting in an increased risk of mortality [46]. Studies of the effects of inhalation antimuscarinics on cardiovascular status have been mixed [47]. Inhalation anticholinergic agents used in chronic obstructive pulmonary disease have been found to aggravate the balance of the autonomic nervous system leading to significantly reduced heart rate recovery following maximal cardiopulmonary exercise [48]. In a longitudinal study of over 3700 nursing home residents with coronary artery disease, the use of anticholinergics was associated with an increased risk of hospitalization and all-cause mortality (hazard ratio 1.71 if the ACB score ≥ 2) [49]. Further, the use of antimuscarinics for urinary incontinence may also be associated with drug-dependent cardiovascular risk. Among these agents, darifenacin has not been associated with an increase in heart rate or QT prolongation because it is M3 selective and it appears to have the best cardiovascular safety profile. Tropsium, on the other hand, may have the highest risk of adverse cardiovascular events. On the basis of these drugs' physiological effects and clinical trials showing increased cardiovascular risk associated with their use, it is best to avoid anticholinergics during the post-myocardial infarction period [50].

8. Practical considerations for the use of anticholinergic agents in older agents

Anticholinergic medications are readily available over-the-counter. First generation antihistamines are available as single ingredients or in multiple symptom cough and cold products. Anticholinergics are marketed as over-the-counter sleep aids and for urinary incontinence [51–54]. A recent study examining older adults' medication decision making and behavior in regards to the use of anticholinergic over-the-counter medications found that while seniors were concerned about adverse drug events, they were not aware of age-related risk associated with the use of anticholinergic medications [55].

Anticholinergic agents are used at end-of-life (EOL) for relief of nausea in those with a vestibular component and more commonly, to provide symptomatic relief of excessive secretions. However, data is lacking to support the use of these drugs for this latter indication [56, 57].

Given the poor risk versus benefit of anticholinergics in older adults, there has been a movement to deprescribe these medications in the elderly. The DEFEAT-polypharmacy was a deprescribing feasibility trial conducted among 46 residential care residents in New Zealand that targeted the use of anticholinergic and sedative medications in older adults. Utilizing peer-reviewed deprescribing guidelines and a collaborative pharmacist-led medication review approach, investigators were able to demonstrate a 0.34 decrease in DBI scores at 6 months. The total number of medications were reduced by 2.13 medications per patient. There was a statistically significant reduction in the number of falls in the past 90 days. There was also a significant improvement in frailty scores. A significant decline was also observed in psychiatric, neurological, autonomic and other adverse events with a decrease in psychiatric adverse events of 1.8 three months after deprescribing and increasing to 2.24 after 6 months; other potential adverse events fell by 2.8 at the end of three months and 4.24 at 6 months post initiation of the deprescribing intervention. Participants also reported lower depression scores after six months. Cognition and quality of life were unchanged [58].

Unfortunately, anticholinergics are sometimes prescribed as part of the prescribing cascade to manage urinary incontinence associated with the use of acetylcholinesterase inhibitors. A population-based retrospective cohort study of 44,884 older adults with dementia conducted in Canada found that there was an increased risk (adjusted hazard ratio 1.55) of subsequently receiving an anticholinergic agent following the initiation of acetylcholinesterase inhibitors [59]. The *Choosing Wisely* campaign, an initiative of the American Board of Internal Medicine Foundation, is designed to promote conversations between clinicians and patients by helping patients choose care that is supported by evidence, not duplicative of other tests or procedures already received, free from harm, and truly necessary. Dialog has started about the use of anticholinergic agents in older adults. In June 2016, the American Academy of Nursing made the following recommendation: "Don't administer "prn" (i.e., as needed) sedative, antipsychotic or hypnotic medications to prevent and/or treat delirium without first assessing for, removing and treating the underlying causes of delirium and using nonpharmacologic delirium prevention and treatment approaches". Anticholinergics are clearly identified as deliriogenic medications [60].

In June 2020, the American Urogynecologic Society (AUS) issued a recommendation stating to "avoid using anticholinergic medication to treat overactive bladder in women older than 70". This recommendation was based on the AUS's concern over the ability of anticholinergic drugs to impair cognition, increase the risk of developing dementia and cause drowsiness and constipation, all potentially detrimental adverse effects in older adults [61].

9. Conclusions

Cholinergic receptors are found throughout the body, but most especially in the CNS. Substances that block these receptors are available both naturally and pharmaceutically. Depending on the location of cholinergic receptors and their subtype, use of anticholinergic medications can result in adverse drug effects in the CNS, the eyes, the exocrine glands, the heart, the GI tract and genitourinary systems and in the skin. Older adults are especially prone to developing adverse drug events from the use of anticholinergics. Easy to use scales are available to assess the burden of anticholinergic agents in the drug regimen. The Beer's List includes drugs that are potentially inappropriate for use in older adults because of their strong anticholinergic properties. Adverse events associated with the use of anticholinergic agents include drowsiness, sedation, cognitive impairment, confusion, delirium, hallucinations, blurred vision, dizziness, falls/fractures, urinary retention, constipation, tachycardia and xerostomia. Anticholinergic drugs have also been associated with an increase in mortality. These agents are involved with numerous drug–drug interactions adding to the anticholinergic burden. They can antagonize the effects of acetylcholinesterase inhibitors, contribute to the development of GI bleeding in patients on oral, solid forms of potassium supplementation and lead to hyperthermia in patients concomitantly receiving a carbonic anhydrase inhibitor. Anticholinergics should not be used by older adults, especially those with narrow angle glaucoma, obstructive uropathy, myasthenia gravis, obstructive GI tract disease and myocardial ischemia. Avoiding prescribing these agents whenever possible is the first step. If they are utilized, it is important for health care professionals to use the lowest doses possible, closely monitor for signs and symptoms of anticholinergic adverse events and to deprescribe as tolerated.

Conflict of interest

The author declares no conflict of interest.

Author details

Donna M. Lisi
PharmD, BCPS, BCGP, BCPP, BCACP, Hackensack Meridian Health, Eatontown, NJ, USA

*Address all correspondence to: drdonnalisi@gmail.com

References

[1] The Editors of Encycloaedia Britannica. Acetylcholine. Encyclopædia Britannica, inc. May 12, 2020. Available from: https://www.britannica.com/science/acetylcholine Accessed 8/15/20.

[2] Rajput H. Effects of *Atropa belladonna* as an anti-cholinergic. *Natural Products Chem Research. 2014, 1,* 1-2. Available from: https://www.longdom.org/open-access/effects-of-atropa-belladonna-as-an-anti-cholinergic-2329-6836.1000104.pdf. Accessed 6/15/20.

[3] Westfall TC, Macarthur H, Westfall DP. Chapter 8. Neurotransmission: the autonomic and somatic motor nervous systems. In: Brunton LL, Hilal-Dandan R, Knollmann BC, editors. Goodman and Gilman's The Pharmacological Basis of Therapeutics. 13th edition. New York; McGraw Hill; 2018. p. 115-47.

[4] Migirov A, Datta AR. Physiology, Anticholinergic reaction. [Updated 2019 Sep 8]. In: StatPearls [Internet]. Treasure Island (FL): StatPearls Publishing; 2020 Jan. Available from: https://www.ncbi.nlm.nih.gov/books/NBK546589/ Accessed 6/20/20.

[5] Tune L, Coyle JT. Serum levels of anticholinergic drugs in treatment of acute extrapyramidal side effects. Arch Gen Psychiatry. 1980;37(3):293-297. doi:10.1001/archpsyc.1980.01780160063007

[6] Tune L, Carr S, Hoag E, Cooper T. Anticholinergic effects of drugs commonly prescribed for the elderly: potential means for assessing risk of delirium. Am J Psychiatry. 1992;149(10):1393-1394. doi:10.1176/ajp.149.10.1393

[7] Ghossein N, Kang M, Lakhkar AD. Anticholinergic medications. [Updated 2020 May 23]. In: StatPearls [Internet]. Treasure Island (FL): StatPearls Publishing; 2020 Jan-. Available from: https://www.ncbi.nlm.nih.gov/books/NBK555893/ Accessed 6/15/20.

[8] Rudolph JL, Salow MJ, Angelini MC, McGlinchey RE. The Anticholinergic Risk Scale and anticholinergic adverse effects in older persons. *Arch Intern Med.* 2008;168(5):508-513. doi:10.1001/archinternmed.2007.106

[9] National Health Service (NHS) Milton Kynes Clinical Commissioning Group. Anticholinergic Cognitive Burden Scale. Available from: http://www.miltonkeynesccg.nhs.uk/resources/uploads/ACB_scale_-_legal_size.pdf Accessed 8/1/20.

[10] Rudolph JL, Salow MJ, Angelini MC, McGlinchey RE. The anticholinergic risk scale and anticholinergic adverse effects in older persons. Arch Intern Med. 2008;168(5):508-513. doi:10.1001/archinternmed.2007.106

[11] Carnahan RM, Lund BC, Perry PJ, Pollock BG, Culp KR. The Anticholinergic Drug Scale as a measure of drug-related anticholinergic burden: associations with serum anticholinergic activity. J Clin Pharmacol. 2006;46(12):1481-1486. doi:10.1177/0091270006292126

[12] Ancelin ML, Artero S, Portet F, Dupuy AM, Touchon J, Ritchie K. Non-degenerative mild cognitive impairment in elderly people and use of anticholinergic drugs: longitudinal cohort study. BMJ. 2006;332(7539):455-459. doi:10.1136/bmj.38740.439664.DE

[13] Ehrt U, Broich K, Larsen JP, Ballard C, Aarsland D. Use of drugs with anticholinergic effect and impact on cognition in Parkinson's disease: a cohort study. J Neurol Neurosurg Psychiatry. 2010;81(2):160-165. doi:10.1136/jnnp.2009.186239

[14] Sittironnarit G, Ames D, Bush AI, et al. Effects of anticholinergic drugs on cognitive function in older Australians: results from the AIBL study. Dement Geriatr Cogn Disord. 2011;31(3):173-178. doi:10.1159/000325171

[15] Bishara D, Harwood D, Sauer J, Taylor DM. Anticholinergic effect on cognition (AEC) of drugs commonly used in older people. Int J Geriatr Psychiatry. 2017;32(6):650-656. doi:10.1002/gps.4507

[16] Kouladjian L, Gnjidic D, Chen TF, Mangoni AA, Hilmer SN. Drug Burden Index in older adults: theoretical and practical issues. Clin Interv Aging. 2014;9:1503-1515. Published 2014 Sep 9. doi:10.2147/CIA.S66660

[17] Hilmer SN, Mager DE, Simonsick EM, et al. A drug burden index to define the functional burden of medications in older people. Arch Intern Med. 2007;167(8):781-787. doi:10.1001/archinte.167.8.781

[18] Salahudeen MS, Duffull SB, Nishtala PS. Anticholinergic burden quantified by anticholinergic risk scales and adverse outcomes in older people: a systematic review. BMC Geriatr. 2015;15:31. Published 2015 Mar 25. doi:10.1186/s12877-015-0029-9 Available from: https://bmcgeriatr.biomedcentral.com/track/pdf/10.1186/s12877-015-0029-9 Accessed 6/15/20. Accessed 6/10/20

[19] Tune LE. Perspective: Serum anticholinergic drug level determinations after 30 Years. Am J Geriatr Psychiatry. 2016;24(12):1189-1190. doi:10.1016/j.jagp.2016.08.021

[20] Beers MH, Ouslander JG, Rollingher I, Reuben DB, Brooks J, Beck JC. Explicit criteria for determining inappropriate medication use in nursing home residents. UCLA Division of Geriatric Medicine. Arch Intern Med. 1991;151(9):1825-1832.

[21] Marcum ZA, Hanlon JT. Commentary on the new American Geriatric Society Beers criteria for potentially inappropriate medication use in older adults. Am J Geriatr Pharmacother. 2012;10(2):151-159. doi:10.1016/j.amjopharm.2012.03.002

[22] By the 2019 American Geriatrics Society Beers Criteria® Update Expert Panel. American Geriatrics Society 2019 Updated AGS Beers Criteria® for Potentially Inappropriate Medication Use in Older Adults. J Am Geriatr Soc. 2019;67(4):674-694. doi:10.1111/jgs.15767

[23] Broderick ED, Metheny H, Crosby B. Anticholinergic toxicity. [Updated 2020 Jun 22]. In: StatPearls [Internet]. Treasure Island (FL): StatPearls Publishing; 2020 Jan-. Available from: https://www.ncbi.nlm.nih.gov/books/NBK534798/ Accessed 6/15/20.

[24] Sura SD, Carnahan RM, Chen H, Aparasu RR. Prevalence and determinants of anticholinergic medication use in elderly dementia patients. Drugs Aging. 2013;30(10):837-844. doi:10.1007/s40266-013-0104-x

[25] Egberts A, Moreno-Gonzalez R, Alan H, et al. Anticholinergic drug burden and delirium: a systematic review. J Am Med Direct Ass. 2020. Available from: https://doi.org.10.1016/j.jamda/2020.04.019 Accessed 8/1/20

[26] Pasina L, Colzani L, Cortesi L, et al. Relation between delirium and Anticholinergic Drug Burden in a cohort of hospitalized older patients: an observational study. Drugs Aging. 2019;36(1):85-91. doi:10.1007/s40266-018-0612-9

[27] Dyer AH, Murphy C, Segurado R, et al. for the NILVAD Study Group. Is ongoing anticholinergic burden associated with greater cognitive decline and dementia severity in mild

to moderate Alzheimer's disease?. J Gerontol A Biol Sci Med Sci. 2020;75(5):987-994. doi:10.1093/gerona/glz244

[28] Neal SR, Wood AD, Ablett AD, et al. Anticholinergic burden in middle-aged women and recurrent falls in later life: findings from the Aberdeen prospective osteoporosis screening study (APOSS). Ther Adv Drug Saf. 2020;11:2042098620929852. Published 2020 May 27. doi:10.1177/2042098620929852 Available from: https://www.ncbi.nlm.nih.gov/pmc/articles/PMC7273562/pdf/10.1177_2042098620929852.pdf Accessed 6/20/20

[29] Ali, S., Peterson, G.M., Bereznicki, L.R. et al. Association between anticholinergic drug burden and mortality in older people: a systematic review. Eur J Clin Pharmacol . 2020; 76: 319-335. Available from: https://doi.org/10.1007/s00228-019-02795-x Accessed 6/20/20

[30] Horn JP, Hansten P. Cholinergic-anticholinergic drug interactions. Pharm Times. 2005; 71(8): 46.

[31] Donepezil (Aricept®) Prescribing Information. Woodcliff Lakes, NJ; Eisai Pharmaceutical. December 2018.

[32] Galantamine (Razadyne®) Prescribing Information. Titusville, NJ; Janssen Pharmaceutical. March 2020.

[33] Rivastigmine (Exelon®) Prescribing Information. East Hanover, NJ; Novartis Pharmaceutical. December 2018.

[34] Atropine and potassium chloride. Drugs.com Drug Interactions Checker. Available from: https://www.drugs.com/drug-interactions/atropine-with-potassium-chloride-280-0-1912-0.html?professional=1 Accessed 8/15/20

[35] Atropine and potassium citrate. Drugs.com Drug Interactions Checker. Available from: https://www.drugs.com/drug-interactions/atropine-with-potassium-citrate-280-0-1914-0.html?professional=1 Accessed 8/15/20

[36] Zarowitz BJ. Oral solid potassium chloride and anticholinergic medications: a new drug interaction for an old drug?. Geriatr Nurs. 2006;27(6):329-333. doi:10.1016/j.gerinurse.2006.10.015

[37] Atropine and topiramate. Drugs.com Drug Interactions Checker. Available from: https://www.drugs.com/drug-interactions/atropine-with-topiramate-280-0-2216-0.html?professional=1 Accessed 8/15/20

[38] Atropine and zonisamide. Drugs.com Drug Interactions Checker. Available from: https://www.drugs.com/drug-interactions/atropine-with-zonisamide-280-0-2334-0.html?professional=1 Accessed 8/15/20

[39] Atropine and morphine. Drugs.com Drug Interactions Checker. Available from: https://www.drugs.com/drug-interactions/atropine-with-morphine-280-0-1656-0.html?professional=1 Accessed 8/15/20

[40] Atropine drug interactions. Drugs.com Drug Interactions Checker. Available from: https://www.drugs.com/drug-interactions/atropine-index.html?filter=2 Accessed 8/15/20

[41] Wu A, Khawaja AP, Pasquale LR, Stein JD. A review of systemic medications that may modulate the risk of glaucoma. Eye (Lond). 2020;34(1):12-28. doi:10.1038/s41433-019-0603-z

[42] Atropine disease interactions. Drugs.com Drug Interactions Checker. Available from: https://www.drugs.com/disease-interactions/atropine.html#:~:text=Anticholinergics%20(Includes%20atropine)%20%E2%86%94%20obstructive%20

uropathy&text=In%20general%2C%20the%20use%20of,occur%20and%20may%20require%20catheterization. Accessed 8/15/20

[43] Jowkar A. Myasthenia Gravis. Medscape. Available from: https://emedicine.medscape.com/article/1171206-overview Accessed 6/15/20

[44] Anonymous. Learning Radiology. Colonic pseudo-obstruction. Available from: http://www.learningradiology.com/archives2011/COW%20465-Ogilvies/ogilviescorrect.htm Accessed 6/15/20

[45] Klabunde RA. Cardiovascular pharmacology concepts- Atropine (muscarinic receptor antagonist). Available from: https://www.cvpharmacology.com/antiarrhy/atropine Accessed 6/15/20

[46] Myint PK, Fox C, Kwok CS, Luben RN, Wareham NJ, Khaw KT. Total anticholinergic burden and risk of mortality and cardiovascular disease over 10 years in 21,636 middle-aged and older men and women of EPIC-Norfolk prospective population study. Age Ageing. 2015;44(2):219-225. doi:10.1093/ageing/afu185

[47] Dweik RA. Role of anticholinergic therapy in COPD. Up-to- Date.com Available from: https://www.uptodate.com/contents/role-of-anticholinergic-therapy-in-copd?search=Anticholinergic%20therapy%20in%20copd&source=search_result&selectedTitle=1~150&usage_type=default&display_rank=1#H91301605 Literature review current through: Jul 2020. | This topic last updated: Jun 06, 2019. Accessed 8/15/20

[48] Yuan W, Nie S, Wang H, Xu Q, Jia N. Anticholinergics aggravate the imbalance of the autonomic nervous system in stable chronic obstructive pulmonary disease. BMC Pulm Med. 2019;19(1):88. Published 2019 May 9. doi:10.1186/s12890-019-0848-0 Available from: https://bmcpulmmed.biomedcentral.com/track/pdf/10.1186/s12890-019-0848-0 Accessed 8/15/20

[49] Vetrano DL, La Carpia D, Grande G, et al. Anticholinergic medication burden and 5-Year risk of hospitalization and death in nursing home elderly residents with coronary artery disease. J Am Med Dir Assoc. 2016;17(11):1056-1059. doi:10.1016/j.jamda.2016.07.012

[50] Anonymous. Antimuscarinic therapy and cardiac safety in older patients with overactive bladder: what clinicians need to Kkow. Consultant360. 2007 February; 15 Supplement 02A. Available from: https://www.consultant360.com/articles/antimuscarinic-therapy-and-cardiac-safety-older-patients-overactive-bladder-what-clinicians Accessed 6/20/20

[51] Rochon PA. Drug prescribing for older adults. Up-to-Date. https://www.uptodate.com/contents/drug-prescribing-for-older-adults#H6. Literature review current through: Jul 2020. | This topic last updated: Jun 08, 2020. Available from: https://www.uptodate.com/contents/drug-prescribing-for-older-adults Accessed 8/1/20

[52] Gray SL, Anderson ML, Dublin S, et al. Cumulative use of strong anticholinergics and incident dementia: a prospective cohort study. *JAMA Intern Med.* 2015;175(3):401-407. doi:10.1001/jamainternmed.2014.7663

[53] Coggins MD. Antihistamine risks. Today's Geriatric Medicine. 2013; 6(2): 6. Available from: https://www.todaysgeriatricmedicine.com/archive/0313p6.shtml Accessed 8/1/20

[54] Albert SM, Roth T, Vitiello M, et al. Over-the-counter sleep aids. Today's Geriatric Medicine. 2016.

9(2): 20. Available from: https://www.todaysgeriatricmedicine.com/archive/MA16p20.shtml Accessed 8/1/20

[55] Holden RJ, Srinivas P, Campbell NL, et al. Understanding older adults' medication decision making and behavior: A study on over-the-counter (OTC) anticholinergic medications. Res Social Adm Pharm. 2019;15(1):53-60. doi:10.1016/j.sapharm.2018.03.002

[56] Albert RH. End-of-Life Care: common symptoms. Am Fam Physician. 2017;95(6):356-361.

[57] Kolb H, Snowden A, Stevens E. Systematic review and narrative summary: Treatments for and risk factors associated with respiratory tract secretions (death rattle) in the dying adult. J Adv Nurs. 2018;74(7):1446-1462. doi:10.1111/jan.13557

[58] Ailabouni N, Mangin D, Nishtala PS. DEFEAT-polypharmacy: deprescribing anticholinergic and sedative medicines feasibility trial in residential aged care facilities. Int J Clin Pharm. 2019;41(1):167-178. doi:10.1007/s11096-019-00784-9

[59] Gill SS, Mamdani M, Naglie G, et al. A prescribing cascade involving cholinesterase inhibitors and anticholinergic drugs. *Arch Intern Med.* 2005;165(7):808-813. doi:10.1001/archinte.165.7.808

[60] American Academy of Nursing. Don't administer "prn" (i.e., as needed) sedative, antipsychotic or hypnotic medications to prevent and/or treat delirium without first assessing for, removing and treating the underlying causes of delirium and using nonpharmacologic delirium prevention and treatment approaches. Choosing Wisely. June 12, 2016. Available from: https://www.choosingwisely.org/clinician-lists/nursing-medications-to-prevent-or-treat-delirium/ Accessed 8/15/20

[61] American Urogynecologic Society. Avoid using anticholinergic medication to treat overactive bladder in women older than 70. Choosing Wisely. June 24, 2020. Available from: https://www.choosingwisely.org/clinician-lists/augs-avoid-using-anticholinergic-medication-to-treat-overactive-bladder-in-women-older-than-70/ Accessed 8/15/20

Chapter 9

Not All Rehabilitation is Physical Therapy

Abel Toledano-González

Abstract

When we are faced with problems that have arisen or are secondary to a particular pathology, the first thing that comes to mind is that we should go to the psychologist, social worker or physiotherapist, but what about functionality and personal autonomy? How can this influence our daily life activities? The occupational therapist, unfortunately little known or undervalued, plays an essential role in this type of situation and especially in work with the elderly.

Keywords: rehabilitation, occupational therapy, personal autonomy, geriatrics, functionality, daily life

1. Introduction

During the last few years, Gerontology and Geriatrics have experienced a great impulse from both classical research and the growing interest in the processes of population ageing in the search for quality of life and personal independence in the last phases of life [1].

Cognitive abilities or skills such as memory, evocation or recovery of information (sensory, short or long term) or contrary as the loss of efficiency in the performance of the activity, secondary to any of the functions mentioned above, can cause further deterioration of the subject that reduces both the quality of life and their level of autonomy [2].

Active ageing as we know it today emerged in the sixties and seventies with a focus on life satisfaction related to the activity people were carrying out, requiring new roles to compensate for those lost and in turn a feeling of being active and participating in society [3].

2. Care in geriatrics and gerontology

It is difficult to choose the appropriate care resource for the person, considering the intervention process and the level of care based on the factors or means available, which can sometimes influence the final treatment and, therefore, the planning, methods and techniques key to the treatment goals set.

Regarding rehabilitation, both the functional recovery, extension or time of the intervention and the quality of it are based on the patient's premorbid state, the evolution or prognosis of the pathology and the involvement of the social environment [4].

Starting with the preparation of a patient profile, gathering as much information as possible from family members, the user and other professionals, we complete what we call an occupational history. This history provides us with information about the patient's lifestyle, interests and evolution, which allows us to identify the activities that are most appropriate for the patient's condition and tastes, with the aim of involving the user during the treatment or operation in order to maintain both their attention and their predisposition towards the objectives previously set, whether these objectives are established or agreed upon with the patient.

Taking into account that multipathology, common both in this type of population either by age or symptoms, usually accompanies the geriatric population, achieving greater independence or autonomy prior to the current situation is a difficult task, since the body's own systems are not as they were in years or states prior to the current one, so in some cases it is only possible to partially recover the systems or alleviate this deficit with the use of external tools or support products that allow users to bridge the gap with their previous state, allowing them to perform the activity in the most standardized way possible [5, 6].

The training and adequacy of an adequate care team is key to offering an optimal comprehensive geriatric service, which allows the realization and design of an appropriate and personalized intervention plan according to the characteristics of the user. The difficulty of intervening in a geriatric patient requires the inclusion of different disciplines that can complete all the areas in which the patient may present some type of problem (physical, functional, psychological and social).

The fact that the multidisciplinary team is an important part of the user's approach allows us to identify different points of view on the same areas of intervention, being able to exchange information and work towards a common goal [7].

2.1 Occupational therapy and activity

According to the World Federation of Occupational Therapy (WFOT), occupational therapy is defined as a profession that promotes health and well-being through the use of occupation as a means. The main objective is to encourage people to become independent in their activities in order to improve their participation. These activities allow the user to increase the independent functions that he or she maintains, enhance development, prevent disability, and improve independence and quality of life [8]. Through this objective, it allows the development of performance components necessary to carry out the activities without problems based on the therapeutic use of the activity with purpose during the intervention process [9].

Therefore, occupational therapy can be understood as the profession that deals with through a meaning or directed to a purpose, with the activity as a base, evaluate, facilitate, restore and maintain a function. Depending on the objectives set by the occupational therapist, it can provide the means to enhance strength, promote social action, stimulate cognitive functions, etc. [10] (**Figure 1**).

The activity is a set of actions carried out with the aim of meeting the goals of an operational program. It consists of the execution of processes and tasks, using certain human, economic and material resources assigned to the final activity.

Such action must maintain or contemplate a meaning for the individual or a feeling of competence that will be important to engage the user during the therapeutic process and thus produce positive feedback.

On the other hand, the activity (meaningful for the user) can be graduated or adapted to facilitate or promote the full implementation of the activity [11].

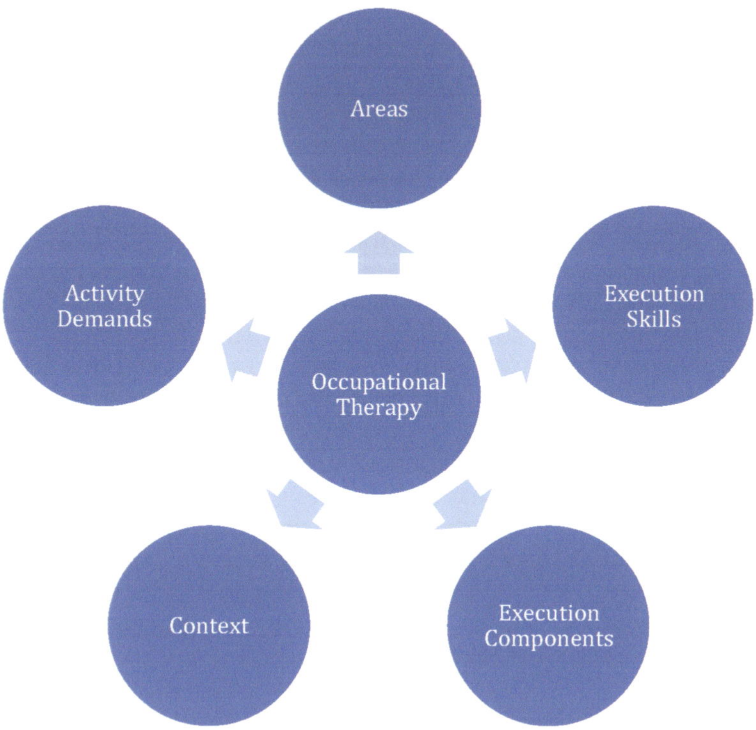

Figure 1.
AOTA Model 2014 [6].

Depending on the focus or direction you want to take on the type of activity to be used, level of demand or qualities needed to carry it out, so during the previous design a challenge will be proposed that is sufficiently important to motivate your positive participation in the activity.

Associated with the sense and meaning that human activity should carry about emotional well-being, Csikszentmihalyi proposes a different way of understanding activities adapted to the different capacities of people, providing that sensation of flow or letting go, thus giving birth to the "Flow Theory". This emotional experience after carrying out the activity allows to report during the participation a positive and pleasant feeling while carrying out [12].

This theory is developed around the search for optimal user experiences during the performance of activities, based on previous experience, skills and abilities in a balance between the possibility of realization and the ability to act of the subject.

This level of challenge or demand for the activity must be appropriate to their capacities/skills, encouraging, as mentioned above, their participation, promoting positive feedback and a balance between the patient's demands and skills.

Happiness is defined as the basis of the quality of life of people, but it also requires what one does to be happy, developing goals that bring meaning to our lives, giving a feeling of satisfaction for something well done through the construction of one's own goals, development of potential, intrinsic motivation enjoying the performance of the activity and motivation in its completion [13]. On the other hand, this lack of time or feeling causes adverse feelings such as stress, increased social concerns or even decreased physical and mental health.

The Flow Theory cites the conditions in which an activity can be considered therapeutic, which are when commitment and concentration are allowed and the user has the necessary tools to carry it out.

Another theory related to the application or use of activities is the DOiT Model (Dynamic Occupation in Time Model) developed by Larson. This model proposes a continuous development of the activity and its skills related to the passing of time together with the subjective experience (Well-Being). The dynamic participation of the therapists in the selection of the activities allows to suggest different forms and strategies of approach, looking for the most positive experience during the time of accomplishment (**Figure 2**) [14].

A greater commitment in developing activities will awaken a feeling of competence, causing a diversion of your energy towards those things in which you show the greatest interest, the greatest need and therefore the search for feedback after completion.

This commitment is generated once the patient actively participates in the activity, Flaherty [15] proposes that some activities provoke an emotional response or interest that leads to commitment, but at the same time these are influenced by their capacities and abilities, past experiences, etc.

If we base ourselves on what Flaherty mentions, quality of life is a determining factor in the individual's interest in participating, in the emotional response and in the level of commitment to the activity.

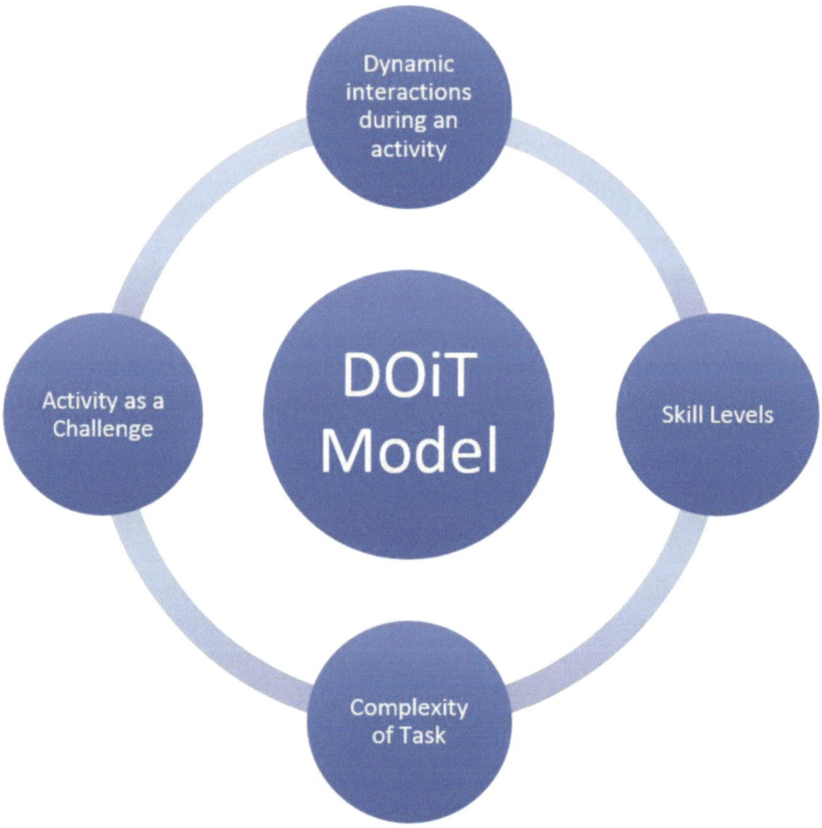

Figure 2.
DOiT Model Interaction. (Extracted from [14]).

2.2 Activities of daily living

Activities of Daily Living (ADL) are those tasks whose purpose is personal self-care with the greatest autonomy and personal independence of the patient. This capacity allows the user to choose or decide for him/herself by making effective use of the freedom [16].

The term coined by the American Occupational Therapy Association (AOTA) brings together all those activities that a person does from the time they get up until they get back up the next day such as: self-care, productivity, leisure and free time. As specified by Romero-Ayuso [10] *"Activities of daily life encompass the most frequent activities performed by a subject, they are related to the familiar, daily, every day, human needs, independence and use of time. Depending on their cognitive complexity and purpose, towards oneself or in relation to the environment, two levels have been established: basic activities and instrumental activities of daily life. The origin of this classification already refers to the importance and need to contemplate the cognitive processes underlying the activity"*

If to all the above we add the aging process, some pathology, the difficulties to maintain that optimal level of autonomy from that moment on increase, so health professionals must focus not only on the disease itself, but also on the repercussions associated with the pathology and the forecast, in order to anticipate and maintain the quality of life of the elderly [17].

3. Psychosocial aspects associated with ageing

Much research highlights aspects that are often associated with older people who are not really older, such as deficits or impairments related to physical or cognitive abilities. The concept associated with active aging defends the opposite, allowing them to maintain healthy and preventive aspects showing a great quality of life that allows them not only to live in their natural environment without problems but to develop as people with identity, roles and maintaining the realization of activities that they usually do in their day to day [18].

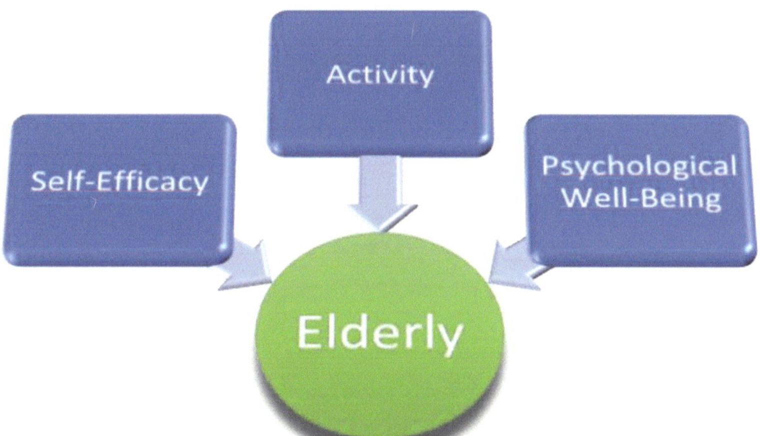

Figure 3.
Psychological factors associated with the elderly (Own elaboration) [19].

On the other hand, it is essential to show the people we work with, in this case older people, why they should carry out these productive or meaningful activities for them, what they can achieve and how it will help them to develop their daily activities in an autonomous and independent way (**Figure 3**).

3.1 The personality

Personality plays a fundamental intrinsic role among the psychological aspects that can influence people to a great extent since, depending on the way they respond, they will carry out the proposed activity in one way or another.

There is an important relationship between activity and life satisfaction, connecting or disconnecting from society as a result of low mood, poor adaptation and other similar emotional disturbances [18].

A peculiarity about the García & González studio [20], is the classification of two groups of people who were more likely to remain active throughout the end of their lives than the other group who showed a tendency to retire early and express a desire to disconnect socially and professionally.

The fact of being active as a formula to maintain personal identity allows and helps the user to enjoy and value positively the time spent, the performance of functions and the promotion of a correct state of mind in this respect.

On the other hand, finding a meaningful activity suitable to one's tastes and personality allows to improve the sense of life, directly affecting the perspective of life, bringing happiness and investing that time in those roles in which they were happy and improving the adaptation of those who remained committed and connected during the last part of their lives [21].

3.2 Psychological well-being

Psychological well-being is defined as the balance between expectations, hope, dreams, achieved or possible realities, expressed with satisfaction and the ability to face vital events in order to adapt [22].

Ryff defines psychological well-being as a multidimensional construct subjectively perceived by the individual defined by the meaning and significance of life for oneself [23].

There are five aspects or areas of psychological well-being:

- Self-acceptance.
- Formation of positive relationships with others.
- Formation of autonomy.
- Mastery of the environment.
- Purpose in life.

Consistent with well-being is self-acceptance, understood by Ryff as the positive attitude towards oneself and one's past, positive relationships as the ability to maintain close relationships with other people, autonomy as self-determination or the ability to make decisions for oneself, mastery of one's environment as the individual's ability to create or choose favourable environments to satisfy needs, purpose in life to provide life with goals, objectives and meaning, and finally purpose in life related to one's potential and personal growth (**Figure 4**).

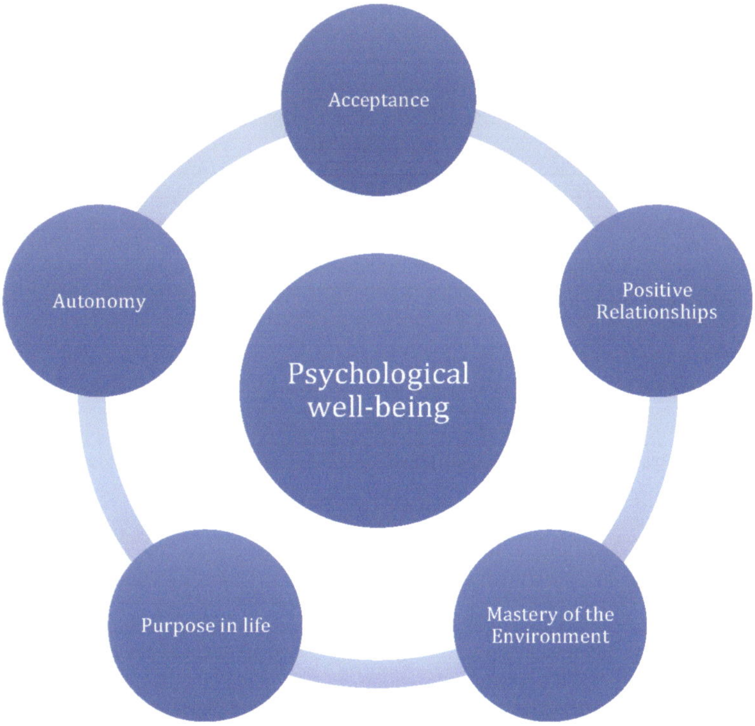

Figure 4.
Element of Psychological Wellbeing (extracted from Ryff and Singer [23]).

3.3 General self-efficacy

A term introduced by Bandura that captures the way one feels, thinks and acts associated with thoughts or as a set of beliefs in one's own abilities to organize and execute actions required to produce achievements or results [24].

In a study on self-efficacy and self-esteem in the Chilean population, the lack of activity was a determining factor in low self-efficacy in young people between 18 and 25 years of age, between 26 and 64 years of age maintained optimal levels of activity and mastery over the performance of roles when they were working, and from 65 years of age onwards after leaving work, it led to greater vulnerability to negative feelings, low social competence and a decrease in personal well-being [19, 25].

Buendia indicated that those older people who unilaterally and voluntarily reduce their social activity by accepting less intense roles and focusing on their inner self, deprive them of a multitude of emotional, physical and financial supports important for their continued personal development [26].

Perceived self-efficacy allows the user to obtain the skills necessary to conclude the desired results with respect to the activity. However, those with higher motivation may choose to undertake activities that are more difficult than those with low motivation, requiring more effort and requiring a sustained commitment.

3.4 Environment and personal independence

One of the most neglected and fundamental factors in the geriatric population is the environment, which can exponentially increase the physical possibilities of the user or increase their inability to carry out an activity, reducing their personal autonomy, a key factor in this population.

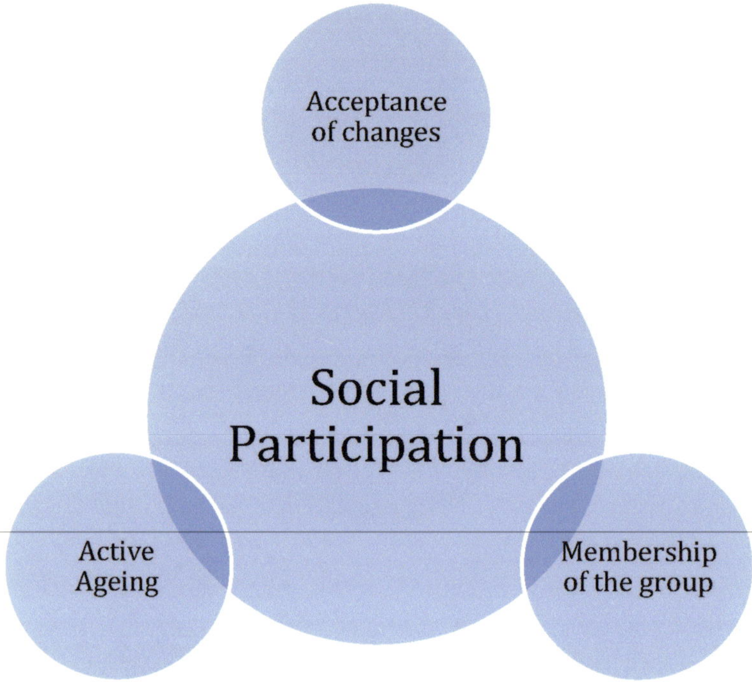

Figure 5.
Interaction of Social Participation and Emotional Well-being. (extracted from [16, 32]).

On many occasions these impossibilities are developed due to the individual's life situation, acting as a barrier to normalized functioning. These excessive incapacities can become real incapacities, weakening the person and accelerating their physiological decline.

A study by Summers allows us to know through non-pathological factors how the role of a psychologist can be decisive in the intervention of functional impairments in the last part of life [27]. This study concluded that the psychological state of the person is a predictor of the degree of disability that the person experiences, taking into account [28].

On the other hand, Rodin [29] in a residential care home for older people carried out a randomized working group distribution based on power of choice and opportunities at a conference. After the conference they were encouraged to accept responsibilities, planning tasks, maintenance of facilities, etc. The other participating group was encouraged to attend talks on attitude, personal assistance, care and personal hygiene.

The results showed that the first group as opposed to the second developed signs of happiness, increased activity, responsiveness, stress reduction, as well as more commitment to the activities offered at the center itself.

If we look at other types of studies such as the one developed by Cummings [30], the passage of age implies a progressive disconnection from the social group, distancing oneself from society and coming to see oneself as a natural part of the ageing process [31] (**Figure 5**).

4. Conclusions

If the characteristics of the people are added together with the possibilities that the environment implies, it can generate or promote a level of activity over the older adult, allowing to give sense to variables or psychological aspects in an intrinsic or extrinsic way in a positive or negative way against a stimulus or activity adapted to their characteristics [33].

Factors such as psychological well-being as a way of accepting oneself and developing one's own potential for personal growth and capacity to face life events, together with self-efficacy as a way of motivating performance, can increase both physical and psychological possibilities in the field of geriatrics.

Finally, as the title of the chapter shows, not everything is physical rehabilitation, since other factors associated with the person must be taken into account, which can play an important role, not only in the predisposition towards a treatment or intervention, but also in the normal development of his/her day-to-day life.

Acknowledgements

To thank Mateo Pulko for giving me the opportunity to participate in this magnificent book through this chapter, to science and all researchers and professionals the task they do with the elderly always looking for their quality of life and wellbeing.

We will all reach that moment one day and we will be happy to know that that professional does everything in his power for us.

The author has received funding by the European Regional Development Fund (2019/7375).

Conflict of interest

The author declares no conflict of interest.

Author details

Abel Toledano-González
Psychology Department, Faculty of Health Sciences, University of Castilla La Mancha, Talavera de la Reina (Toledo), Spain

*Address all correspondence to: atoledanogonzalez@gmail.com

References

[1] Altarriba F. Gerontología: aspectos biopsicosociales del proceso de envejecer. Barcelona: Boixareau Universitaria; 1998.

[2] Jackson J, Carlson M, Mandel D, Zemke R, Clark F. Occupation in lifestyle redesign: The well elderly study occupational therapy program. American Journal of Occupacional Therapy. 1998; 52(5): p. 326-336.

[3] Oddone MJ. Antecedentes teóricos del envejecmiento activo. Informes Envejecimiento en Red. 2013; 4.

[4] Polonio-López B. Valoración geriátrica integral: Papel de la terapia ocupacional. In Durante-Molina P, Pedro-Tarrés P. Terapia Ocupacional en geriatría: principios y práctica. Barcelona: Masson; 2004. p. 29-54.

[5] Legg L, Drummond A, Leonardi-Bee J. Occupational therapy for patients with problems in personal activities of daily living after stroke: a systematic reviez of randomised trials. BMJ. 2007;(335).

[6] Moruno Miralles P, Romero-Ayuso D. Actividades de la vida diaria Barcelona: Masson; 2005.

[7] Calenti M. Gerontología y Geriatría Madrid: Editorial Médica Panamericana; 2010.

[8] Zimmer Z, Hickey T, Searle MS. Activity participation and well-being among older people with arthritis. The Gerontologist. 1995; 35.

[9] Kielhofner G. Respecting both the "occupation" and the "therapy" in our field. American Journal of Occupational Therapy. 2007; 61(4).

[10] Romero-Ayuso D, Moruno Miralles P. Terapia Ocupacional: teoría y técnicas Barcelona: Masson-Elsevier; 2003.

[11] Kronenberg F, Simó Algado S, Pollard N. Terapia ocupacional sin fronteras: aprendiendo el espítiru de supervivientes Buenos Aires: Editorial Médica Panamericana; 2007.

[12] Csikszentmihalhyi M. Fluir. Una psicología de la felicidad Barcelona: Kairós; 2011.

[13] Csikszentmihalhyi M. Aprender a Fluir Barcelona: Kairós; 2009.

[14] Larson EA. The Time of our lives: the experience of temporality in occupation. American Journal of Occupational Therapy. 2004; 71(1).

[15] Flaherty MG. Conceptualizing variation in the experience of time. Social Psychology Quarterly. 1993; 54.

[16] Corregidor-Sánchez I, Gómez Calero C. Área de actividades de la vida diaria. In Corregidor Sánchez I. Terapia Ocupacional en Geriatría. Madrid: Sociedad Geriátrica de Geriatría y Gerontología; 2010.

[17] Rodríguez-Martínez MC, Toledano-González A, Bermnúdez-Bayón U. Terapia Ocupacional en Geriatría Madrid: Síntesis; 2019.

[18] Schmidt V, Leibovich N, Giménez M. Estudio de las propiedades psicométricas de un instrumento para la evaluación de la satisfacción vital global. Calidad de Vida y Salud. 2014; 7.

[19] Toledano-González A, Labajos-Manzanares T, Romero Ayuso D. Occupational Therapy, Self-Efficacy, Well-Being in Older Adults Living in Residential Care Facilities: A Randomized Clinical Trial. Frontiers in Psychology. 2018.

[20] García-Viniegras V, González-Benítez I. La categoría Bienestar Psicológico. Su relación con otras categorías sociales. Revista Cubana de Medicina General Integral. 2000; 16(6).

[21] Hernández-Zamora ZE, Ehrenzeweig-Sánchez Y, Manuel Navarro A. Factores psicológicos, demográficos y sociales asociados al estrés y a la personalidad resistente en adultos mayores. Pensamiento Psicológico. 2010; 5(12).

[22] Molina CJ, Meléndez JC. Bienestar psicológico en envejecimiento de la República Dominicana. Geriatrika. 2006; 22(3).

[23] Ryff CD, Singer BH. Best news yet on the six factor model of well-being. Social Science Research. 2002; 35.

[24] Bandura A. On the Functional Properties of Perceived Self-Efficacy Revisited. Journal of Management. 2012; 38(1).

[25] Aguirre Mas C, Vauro Desiderio R. Autoestima y Autoeficacia de los Chilenos. Ciencia & Trabajo. 2009; 11(32).

[26] Hermida P, Stefani D. La jubilación como un factor de estrés psicosocial. Un análisis de los trabajos científicos de las últimas décadas. Perspectivas en Psicología. 2012; 8(2).

[27] Summers H, Haley E, Reveille J, Alarcón G. Radiographic assessment and psychologic variables as predictors of plan and unfunctional impairment in osteoarthritis of the knee or hip. Arthritis & Rheumatology. 1988; 31(2).

[28] Petrie KJ, Moss Morris R, Gery C, Shaw M. The rlationship of negative affect and perceived sensity to symtom reporting following vaccination. British Journal of Health Psychology. 2004; 9(1).

[29] Rodin J. Health, control and aging. In Baltes MM. Psychology Revivals: The psychology of control and aging. New York: Psychology Press; 2014. p. 139-165.

[30] Cumings E, Henry WE. Growing old: the process of disengagement New York: Basic Book; 1961.

[31] Brodaty H, Altendorf A, Withall A, Sachdev P. Do people become more apathetic as they grow older? A longitudinal study in healthy individuals. Cambridge University Press. 2010; 22(3).

[32] Andonian, L., & MacRae, A. (2011). Well Older Adults within an Urban Context: Strategies to Create and Maintain Social Participation. British Journal of Occupational Therapy, 74(1), 2-11. https://doi.org/10.4276/030802211X12947686093486

[33] Toledano-González A, Labajos-Manzanares T, Romero-Ayuso D. Well-Being, Self-Efficacy and Independence in older adults: A Randomized Trial of Occupacional Therapy. Archives of Gerontology and Geriatrics. 2019.

Section 4

Miscellaneous

Chapter 10

Inappropriate Medication and Perception of Quality of Life in Hospitalized Elderly Patients

Ana Fajreldines, Marisa Bazzano, Belen Beldarrain, Stefanía Barberis and Marcelo Pellizzari

Abstract

Older or elderly adults represent a population exposed to potentially inappropriate prescriptions, since medication is the most widely used intervention. The objective of this work is to analyze the type of medication schemes of the elderly and the relationship with their states of psychological well-being. It is a cross-sectional study. Results: inappropriate prescription is of the order of 16% and the perception of quality of life was 56.8, finding an association between inappropriate prescription and perception of quality of life. Conclusions: The results showed that inappropriate prescription is highly frequent in these patients and that psychological well-being states would be related to this inappropriate prescription.

Keywords: elderly, quality of life, inappropriate prescription of medication

1. Introduction

Worldwide, the proportion of people>60 years of age is increasing faster than that of any other age group. Gender disparities, structural changes in the family and social environment, the number of older people living alone, changes in the burden of disease, drug therapy and the risk of disability, among other factors, indicate the importance of assessing the global health care and the specific problems of this population [1].

There are situations that can cause a worsening of the organic functional capacity of the elderly, such as: medications, illnesses, significant life changes, sudden increase in physical demands. Medications whose risk of adverse drug events (ADE) in the elderly or elderly exceeds expectations of clinical benefits compared to more effective, safe and available alternatives are called potentially inappropriate medications [2].

According to the WHO, quality of life is: "the perception that an individual has of his place in existence, in the context of the culture and value system in which he lives and in relation to his objectives, his expectations, his norms, their concerns. It is a very broad concept that is influenced in a complex way by the physical health of the subject, their psychological state, their level of independence, their social relationships, as well as their relationship with the essential elements of their environment " [3–5]. Due to the aforementioned in this work, the relationship that exists between inappropriate medication and welfare states in the population over 65 years of age is explored.

2. Objectives

To analyze the inappropriate prescription and quality of life of hospitalized elderly according to internationally validated instruments.

3. Materials and methods

Retrospective observational study. The patients included were adults over 64 years hospitalized in the study center. The study was carried out in a highly complex academic hospital in Argentina. The criteria of Screening Tool of Older Person's Prescriptions (STOPP) 2015, [6] of inappropriate prescription of drugs, were used. Polypharmacy was considered to be the simultaneous presence of more than 4 drugs according to the WHO definition [7]. The investigators who analyzed the inappropriate prescriptions were two observers trained in the criteria, both of whom reviewed all cases. Concordance between the two reviewers was assessed with Cohen's Kappa test, obtaining a value of: 0.71 (95% CI 0.65–0.76). The burden of disease was assessed with the Charlson index [8], which predicts mortality and burden of disease according to preceding pathologies. The EURO-QOL 5d [9] scale was used to assess the perception of quality of life that contains 5 dimensions or topics: mobility, personal care, daily activities, pain/ discomfort, anxiety /depression. These topics have three options: - mild, –moderate and -high presence of each topic analyzed. The survey was done in person before discharge and to facilitate the analysis of the results, the questions were divided into three topics: "no problems", "moderate problems", and "serious or serious problems" (coinciding with the three options of each topical). Variables such as sex, age, family life, active patient with current job or in retirement, smoking habit, polypharmacy, among others, were collected. The data were loaded into Excel databases and processed with the SPSS 21 package, IBM®.

4. Results

300 hospitalized patients were studied in the 2016–2018 year. The distribution by sex was: 169 (56.4%) women and 131 (43.6%) men. The mean age was 73.3 + 18.5 years. Median: 69.12.

In the total sample analyzed, 16% (n = 48) showed inappropriate prescription of drugs criteria.

The types of drugs most involved were the following **Table 1**.

The mean well-being of the patients on the scale of 1–100 was 56.8 (SD 23.4), median: 61.7, range: 29–95.

The quality of life scale showed the following **Table 2**.

Of the 300 patients, 143 (47.7%) lived with their family (spouse, children, nephews, grandchildren, etc.), 81 (27%) lived alone or with a non-family caregiver, 76 (25.3%) lived in geriatric.

In an unadjusted multiple binary regression, the association of different variables with the perception of quality of life was the one shown in the following table (**Tables 3** and **4**).

Therapeutical Groups	N	Percentage (IC95%)
Non esteroidal pain relievers	21	43,8 (43,5-44,1)
Oral anticoagulants	16	33,3 (32,9-33,6)
Psychopfarmaceuticals	9	18,7 (18,2-18,9)
Others	2	4,2 (4,1-4,7)

Table 1.
Frequencies by drug type.

Global perception of quality of life	N	Percentage (IC95%)
Without problems	123	41 (40,9-42,3)
With moderate problems	98	32,7 (32,3-32,9)
With serious problems	79	26,3 (26,1-26,8)

Table 2.
The quality of life scale showed the following.

Variable	With PIM	Without PIM	p Value
Without problems	16 (20,25%)	107 (79,75%)	0,001
With moderate problems	38 (38,8%)	60 (61,2%)	0,005
With serius problems	56 (70,8%)	23 (29,2%)	0,002

Table 3.
Quality of life scales with and without inapprorpiate prescription.

Variable	OR (IC 95%)
Inappropriate precsription	1,52 (1,37-2,16)
Active work	1,76(1,16-1,97)
Life in a nursing home	1,89(1,45-2,15)
Female sex	1,98(1,35-2,13)
Polypharmacy	1,11(0,76-1,89)
Age over 80 years	1,13(0,98-2,14)
Severe–moderate pain	1,21(0,96-1,69)
Severe–moderate depression	1,23(0,97-1,34)

Table 4.
Binary multiple regression of different variables with perception of quality of life.

5. Discussion

Overall inappropriate prescribing values are similar by some studies [10, 11].

It is important to note that this study demonstrated a strong association between inappropriate medication with positive STOPP criteria and the perception of a deterioration in quality of life, because a person who receives inappropriate medication increases 2.3 times the chance of perceiving a deterioration in their quality of life.

A systematic review found that the drugs most exclusively included in the inappropriate prescription were non-steroidal anti-inflammatory drugs and benzodiazepines [12]. The review of Mahony [12], it states that the application of the STOPP criteria improves clinical outcomes in multimorbid older people but does not mention the impact it has on quality of life.

Furthermore, it is possible to affirm that there is a relationship between the inappropriate prescription of medication and polypharmacy, female sex, age over 80 years, presence of comorbidities such as pain, anxiety and/or depression.

We have not found studies of quality of life and inappropriate medication. It is important to link the states of well-being with the inappropriate use of medications to know other impacts on the public health of this population segment.

6. Conclusions

After carrying out this work, it is concluded that aging is characterized by a series of extremely individualized physiological, psychological and social factors, that older adults represent a risk group with a higher degree of vulnerability to drugs. The most commonly used medications are pain relievers, oral anticoagulants and psychotropic drugs. We have shown that there is a close relationship between the medication administered in the elderly and the perception of quality of life. Therefore, it is essential that their prescription be carried out individually, taking into account the social and family context of the patient.

Acknowledgements

To Eduardo Schnitzler, MD

Conflicts of interest

The authors declare no conflict of interest.

Author details

Ana Fajreldines*, Marisa Bazzano, Belen Beldarrain, Stefanía Barberis and Marcelo Pellizzari
Aleman Hospital, Austral University Hospital, Buenos Aires, Argentina

*Address all correspondence to: fajreldinesa@gmail.com

References

[1] Motter RF, Soder Fritzen J, Hilmer S, Vieira Paniz E, Vieira Paniz VM. Potentially inappropriate medication in the elderly: a systematic review of validated explicit criteria. Review Eur J Clin Pharmacol. 2018 Jun; 74(6):679-700. doi: 10.1007/s00228-018-2446-0. Epub 2018 Mar 27.

[2] O'Mahony D. STOPP/START criteria for potentially inappropriate medications in older people: origin and progress Review Expert Rev Clin Pharmacol. 2020 Jan;13(1):15-22. doi: 10.1080/17512433.2020.1697676. Epub 2019 Nov 30.

[3] Guil Sánchez J. Adequacy of Drug Prescriptions in Elderly Patients Admitted to a Convalescence Unit According Beers Criteria. Rev Calid Asist Nov-Dec 2013;28(6):391-3. doi: 10.1016/j.cali.2013.05.004. Epub 2013

[4] WHOQOL GROUP. The World Health Organization Quality of life assessment (WHOQOL). Position Paper from the World Health Organization. Soc. Sci. Med. 1995; 41(10):1.403-1.409.

[5] Brombo G, Bianchi L, Maietti E, Malacarne F, Corsonello A, et al. Web site of WHO World Health Organization. http://www.who.int/mediacentre/news/releases/2014/world-health-statistics-2014/es

[6] Pendlebury ST, Lovett NG, Smith SC, Dutta N, Bendon C, Lloy-Levery A et al. Observational, longitudinal, study of delirium in consecutive unselected acute medical admissions: age specific rate and associated factors mortality and re admission. BMJ Open 2015, Nov 16;5(11):e007808 doi101136/bmjopm-2015 007808.

[7] Brombo G, Bianchi L, Maietti E, Malacarne F, Corsonello A, et al. Association of Anticholinergic Drug Burden with Cognitive and Functional Decline Over Time in Older Inpatients: Results from the CRIME Project.Drugs Aging. 2018 Oct;35(10):917-924. doi: 10.1007/s40266-018-0584-9.

[8] Charlson ME, Pompei P, Ales KL. A new method of classifying prognostic comorbidity in longitudinal studies: development and validation. J Chronic Dis 1987; 40:373-83.

[9] EuroQol group. EuroQol – a new facility for the measurement of health-related quality of life. Health Policy 1990; 16: 199-208.

[10] Li H, Pu S, Liu Q, Huang X, Kuang J, et al. Potentially inappropriate medications in Chinese older adults: The beers criteria compared with the screening tool of older persons'prescriptions criteria. Geriatr Gerontol Int. 2017;17(11):1951-1958. doi: 10.1111/ggi.12999.

[11] Achterhof AB, Rozsnyai Z, Reeve E, Jungo KT, Floriani C, Poortvliet RKE, et al. Potentially inappropriate medication and attitudes of older adults towards deprescribing. Streit S.PLoS One. 2020 Oct 26;15(10):e0240463. doi: 10.1371/journal.pone.0240463. eCollection 2020.

[12] Todd A, Esposo A, Andrew I, Pearson SA, Lindsey L, Holmes H. Inappropriate prescription of preventive drugs in patients with life-limiting diseases: a systematic review. BMJ Support Palliat Care. 2017. 7 (2): 113-121. doi: 10.1136 / bmjspcare-2015-000941. Epub 2016.

Chapter 11

Motivation and Social Support Received in Elderly Care: The Case of Geriatric Palliative Caregivers

Wilfred Luis Clamor

Abstract

This study describes the experiences on geriatric palliative care of 12 caregivers in Metro Manila. This study looks on the variation of experiences on motivation and social support in caregiving. This study used a qualitative-descriptive research design and involved key informant interviews of caregivers as a research method. Informants were selected through a non-probability sampling technique specifically through a purposive-convenient sampling. Caregivers cite several of motivations for caregiving. Reasons mentioned are identified to be either intrinsic motivation or extrinsic motivation. Intrinsic motivation being cited are emphatic reasons which include framing patient as family; emotional reasons such as emotional attachment; and cognitive reasons which refers to gaining knowledge in caregiving. Extrinsic motivations by caregivers are incentive reasons which include monetary gains; and negative reinforcements such as institutional punishments. In terms of social support received, caregivers mentioned different sources and functions of support they receive. Caregivers cite two types of social support structure or sources, proximal social support and institution based support. For social support function, responses are categorized into intangible and tangible support.

Keywords: geriatric healthcare and management, geriatric palliative caregiving, motivation, social support structure, social support function

1. Introduction

In the past decade, the caregiving profession is known to continue to increase because of the fast growth of the aging population [1]. In that sense, caregivers are high in demand because of the present global situation most especially those who are formal or professional workers and volunteers under long term facilities. Caregivers are individuals who tend to express caregiving behaviors that are required in their job description. Moreover, caregiving is a phenomenon that is increasingly studied by the medical and social sciences field [2]. Caregiving is an act of tending and caring for other individual with a problematic health condition or impairment in a daily basis.

Caregivers experience different situations doing geriatric palliative care. In the past literatures, various studies found different factors that may influence doing palliative care to elderly individuals. A study by Pearlin and Schooler [3], found that personal control and mastery has been a significant factor that shapes the caregiver's experience in doing caregiving. With personal mastery, an individual has the capability to manipulate their actions hence overcomes different challenges. In the caregiver's perspective, they may be able to experience more positive experiences because they can control and manipulate their actions [4, 5].

In sociology, focuses on the global perspective of the concept of caregiving through caregivers, caregiver roles, and characteristics of caregivers as well as their motivations and social networks. Also, caregiving is studied through groups of caregivers or health care professionals tending to individuals who are in need of care. Caregiving in the field of sociology is studied through the experiences of caregivers from groups and organizations such as family, neighbors, health care institutions, as well as individuals affiliated with religious institutions [6]. All in all, sociologists focus on the influences of behaviors such as motivation as well as social networks of caregivers.

In recent studies, it is found that motivation plays a vital role among caregivers in doing palliative care towards elderly patients. Motivation is defined to be reinforcements for an individual to express a certain kind of behavior [7]. In the past, motivation is studied in the field of social psychology. Various theories explained with certain motivations, individuals manifest a particular behavior. Motivations are divided into two types: intrinsic and extrinsic motivation. Intrinsic motivations are reinforcements that are internal in nature. One example of intrinsic reinforcement is having altruistic motivation. According to a study by Hyde, Harris, and Boaden [8], health care workers manifest altruism in dealing with their patients. Altruistic motivation is having a voluntary mindset intended to help and increase another's welfare because the attitude of being concerned for others [9]. Moreover, it is a motivation that seeks to overcome the feeling of sympathy towards individuals who needs help [10]. According to a study by Bhatti and Qureshi [11], health care workers are motivated by the desire to help and take on a useful activity. In the case of geriatric palliative caregiving, caregivers feel the sense of helping their elderly patients without any compensation in return. This is mostly seen among voluntary workers in nursing homes run by religious organizations.

Another theory to explain the intrinsic motivations of doing geriatric palliative caregiving is Selective Investment Theory (SIL). This theory talks about social bonds or close relationship provides motivation that makes individuals suppress their own personal goals if need to prioritize the overall well-being of the other [7]. Moreover, the theory gives emphasis on the role of having close relationships in meeting the needs of other individuals. In recent literatures, caregivers' witness their patients' life at nursing homes hence makes them attached. With attachment, caregivers tend to care more and give more importance to their patients rather than their personal life.

Emotional motivation is also found to be an effective reinforcement for individuals. In a study by Carlo and Randall [10], the feeling of empathy triggers an individual to act or behave in a certain way because of strong emotions. It evokes mostly individuals who are easily affected by people who manifest emotional behaviors. For health care workers, a feeling of empathy urges them to work hard to do pain management on their elderly patients.

Social desirability is a motivation that evokes individuals to behave in a certain way because of social pressure and norms [12]. Individuals are more likely to express caregiving behavior when being observed by their superiors. Also, caregivers feel pressure from their supervisors in order to accomplish their tasks and jobs in doing geriatric palliative caregiving. It is a norm that caregivers must do caregiving duties and nothing else. This reinforces caregivers to tend to their task and normal work. Also, health care workers are motivated to work harder when it is on the motive of desiring a gain of approval and respect from other people most especially their superiors [10].

For extrinsic kinds of motivation, the most frequently used in the health care sector is compensation and punishment. It is found that both are effective tools for reinforcing individuals to comply with their job description. However according to Kreps [13], "providing extrinsic incentives for workers can be counterproductive, because it may destroy the workers' intrinsic motivation (p. 359)." In that sense, extrinsic motivation may not be truly effective in reinforcing individuals because it is found to be inefficient.

Access to social support is also a proximal factor that influences the experiences of caregivers in doing geriatric palliative caregiving. Social support is an available assistance from other people and it is also a coping resource used by individuals [14]. Moreover, it talks about received encouragement and assistance by individuals from other people. According to Albrecht and Adelman [15], social support is defined to be a "verbal and nonverbal communication between recipients and providers that reduces uncertainty about the situation, the self, the other, or the relationship, and functions to enhance a perception of personal control in one's life experience (p. 18)".

Social support can be a discourse between two entities. This concept is understood to be given or received. On one hand, social support is an act or behavior that an individual that is to be given to another individual. On the other hand, it is also an act that an individual receives from another individual [16]. Social support can be measured in two categories. One category is called structural support or social integration. It measures the quantity or the extent of which an individual is connected to a social network [17]. This category measures the size, frequency, or density of a social network of an individual [18]. Another category is called functional social support. This measures the quality or functional aspects of social support. It looks on the roles of the social network provides. Functions such as emotional support which focuses on the affect and emotional nurture provided by sources of social support; esteem support which focuses on bolstering an individual to handle a difficult situations; network support which focuses on the affirmation of an individual as a part of a social network; informational support which focuses on which focuses on a the communication that gives insightful information; and tangible support which focuses physical assistance and support [19].

According to Kaufman, Kosberg, Leeper, and Tang [20] having good social support causes positive behavior in doing health care management specifically in the spiritual aspect of geriatric palliative caregiving. Moreover, with good social support, the caregiving job becomes less challenging and burdensome because it is known as a coping resource used by caregivers [14]. However, the caregiving experience becomes challenging and burdensome because of factors such as lack of emotional support from colleagues and peers, social isolation, and inadequate social activities about coping [21].

Support also comes from different sources. It may come from colleagues, peers, and most especially family. Research found that lack of family support has been found to "correlate with high levels of physical as well as psychological exhaustion, with many caregivers reporting that their social support decreases over time" [14].

There may be a lot of studies about motivation and social support, however very limited studies were seen focusing on the variation of motivations and social support structure and functions of geriatric palliative caregivers in the Philippines. With that, the objective of this study is to describe various motivations and social support experiences of caregivers in geriatric palliative caregiving.

2. Methodology

This study used a qualitative-descriptive research design. This study describes the motivation and social support experiences of professional caregivers tending to elderly patients under intensive care. This study involved key informant interviews of caregivers as a research method. In addition, this involved a face-to-face interview as a research technique.

The population of this study involved professional caregivers employed in a private nursing home in Metro Manila. This study involved 12 key informants as sample. This study utilized a non-probability sampling technique. Key informants are chosen through a purposive-convenient sampling. To be eligible for the interview, the sample should fit the specific selection criteria: 1) Must have an experience doing geriatric palliative care; and 2) Has at least one to two years of experience in the caregiving profession.

The voice-recorded in-depth interviews were transcribed, and the data gathered were sorted according to the research problems they addressed. Content analysis was used as data evaluation through an evaluation of the interview transcriptions. The personal and work characteristics of the caregivers were tabulated to present the trends across these phenomena, and similar answers to the interview questions are grouped together. The information were analyzed and presented based on similarities and differences of the themes.

3. Results and discussions

3.1 Personal characteristics

Caregivers in this study are within the age range of 18–35 years old (See **Table 1**). Majority of the caregivers belong to a younger age cohort of 18–23. In terms of educational attainment, most caregivers finished a bachelor's degree in college while other caregivers only finished high school. For religious affiliation, most caregivers

Characteristics	*f*
Age	
18–23	5
24–29	3
30–35	4
Mean	25.83
Educational Attainment	
High School	4
College	8
Civil Status	
Single	9
Married	3
Religions Affiliation	
Catholic	9
Born Again	2
Iglesia ni Cristo	1
Monthly Income	
Php 5000-10,000	9
Php 11,000-15,000	3
Mean	Php 7417

Table 1.
Personal characteristics of caregivers.

are practicing the religion of Catholicism. Caregivers in this study averages to earn a salary of Php7, 417 monthly. Most monthly income of caregivers fall under the category of 5000–10,000 (75.0%) a month while other caregivers receive 11,000–15,000 a month.

Caregivers have various jobs before working at the nursing home. Majority of the informants come from medical and non-care related jobs before entering the career of being a caregiver (See **Table 2**). Medical related jobs involve nursing and pharmacy while non care related jobs pertain to canteen personnel, station personnel, receptionist, and farming. Provision of care delivery related jobs pertain to being a maid/helper, and being a caregiver. Other caregivers are also seen to have no prior work before entering the nursing home.

3.2 Motivations in caregiving

Caregivers have mentioned numerous reasons in doing their jobs. This refers to specific reinforcements that push caregivers while working. The identified motivations for caregiving are classified according to intrinsic motivation and extrinsic motivation (See **Table 3**).

Intrinsic motivation refers to the kind of reinforcements that are internal in nature which focuses on the inherent stimulus of caregivers. Majority of the caregivers cited emphatic reasons as intrinsic motivation. Emphatic reasons such as framing a thought that patients can be family are mentioned. Caregivers stated that this kind of reason is a powerful motivational force in caring for their patients.

Characteristics	*f*
Provision of Care Delivery Related	
Maid/Helper	1
Caregiver	1
Medical Related	
Nurse	3
Pharmacist	1
Non Care Related	
Canteen Personnel	1
Station Personnel	1
Receptionist	1
Farmer	1
No Prior Work	2

Table 2.
Previous jobs of caregivers.

Intrinsic motivation	**Extrinsic motivation**
Empathic Reasons (e.g. framing a thought that patients can be family)	Incentive Reasons (e.g. monetary gains)
Emotional Reasons (e.g. emotional attachment)	Negative Reinforcements (e.g. Institutional punishments)

Table 3.
Motivations in caregiving.

Most caregivers claim that they are more motivated to work because they feel that they are actually caring for their parents or grandparents. This scenario was pointed out by majority of the caregivers.

> *"I even call them my grandparents. I became very close to them because of that. I actually see my grandparents in them. I even treat them as if they are my family"*

> *"I see my parents in them. With that, I more motivated to care for my patients because sometimes I treat them as my own parents."*

This finding is reflected on the idea that Filipinos give utmost priority to close family ties [22]. Caregivers are seen to treat patients as family as a motivation to care for them. Caring for family is a strong motivational force for Filipinos [23]. This emphatic reason is also reflected by Selected Investment Theory (SIL). This theory talks about how social bonds and close relationships drives motivation in giving priority for the betterment of the other [7]. In the case of the result, caregivers having patients as a form of a family provides motivation that makes them suppress personal goals and preferences to promote and give priority on the well-being of the patient.

Emotional reasons are also frequently stated as an intrinsic motivation by most caregivers. This refers to the feeling of concern, care, and love among caregivers to their patients. Most caregivers are found to be assigned to one to two patients in the nursing home. Caring for these patients makes the caregivers attached because there are times that the caregivers want to see their patients happy all the time. Some informants say that they also become sad if their patients are not satisfied or happy. These are true to the majority of the caregivers in the nursing homes.

> *"I am more motivated to care for my patients when I see them sad and depressed. I do not want to see them sick. I feel depressed also when they are not happy."*

Having emotional attachment as a motivation is seen as a protective behavior among caregivers. This attachment is seen also to create a strong bond that urges the caregivers to help and increase their wellbeing due to their situation [24]. This attachment is seen to be a two way relationship between the caregiver and the patient. Caregivers feel accomplished when their patients are happy. Emotional attachment to patients is indeed effective in pursuing their fulfillment and good quality well-being [10].

Another classification for the motivations for caregiving among caregivers is extrinsic motivation. This classification of motivation refers to reinforcements that can be seen or tangible in nature which are in the form of different incentives. Majority of caregivers answer having good salary as an extrinsic motivation. This salary is used to help their families to have financial stability.

In some instances, caregivers admitted to have violated some rules and regulations of the institution. With that, sanctions are also an extrinsic motivation for caregiving. These punishments refer to a deduction in salary, warnings and scolding from their superiors, and even expulsion from the nursing home. In that sense, caregivers are expected to have proper decorum and must follow the rules and regulations of the institutions in order not to be reprimanded by their superiors. Also, some caregivers responded that all must follow their superiors because every caregiver in the institution is to be reprimanded. Caregivers are then motivated to work because they do not want to experience these kinds of institutional punishments. This is true in some caregivers.

"Sometimes we experienced being reprimanded by our superiors. If one gets scolded, everyone receives a penalty that is why all of us are motivated to work in order for us to not experience those punishments."

Negative reinforcement could lead to counterproductive workplace environment among workers according to the study of Kreps [13]. However, based on the results mentioned, caregivers are motivated to work harder not to be reprimanded and experience negative reinforcement. With that, these institutional punishments can be very effective in managing workers in an organization. It is seen as an effective tool for workers to comply with their job roles in the company or organization.

3.3 Social support received by caregivers

While tending to their patients, caregivers receive different kinds of encouragement from different social actors. Social support ensures that caregivers are motivated and satisfied with their current situation. Social support received by caregivers is classified into two categories, social support structure and social support function.

3.3.1 Social support structure

Caregivers receive different kinds of support from different social entities. Social support is a coping resource as well as assistance coming from other individuals [14]. Social support structure refers to the people or social actors supporting caregivers in doing their job. According to Wills [17], it measures the quantity or the extent of which an individual is connected to a social network. This category of social support measures the size, frequency, or density of a social network of an individual [18]. The identified social support structure is classified according to proximal social support and institution based support (See **Table 4**).

Caregivers are mentioned to be surrounded by individuals in the nursing homes. These individuals are seen to encourage the caregivers in doing their job. This refers to proximal social support. Majority of caregivers responded that their colleagues are the most proximal in terms of social support. The colleagues of the caregivers are seen to be a significant support by means of encouragement and provision. Also, caregivers and their colleagues converse about their personal and work related problems. This conversation sets as a way of supporting one another to resolve certain kinds of personal and work related problems. According a female caregiver,

"Most of the time, my colleagues and I talk about our problems. We then help each other at the same time."

Proximal social support	Institution based support
Support from colleagues (e.g. co-workers & subordinates)	Support from superiors (e.g. owners and supervisors)
Support from patients (e.g. elderly patients)	Support from patient's family (e.g. children of the patient)
Support from family (e.g. parents and siblings)	

Table 4.
Social support structure.

The patients of the caregivers are also seen to give social support. Caregivers admitted that their patients also tend to encourage and support them. While caregivers are tending to the needs of their patients, it is also seen that these health care workers converse with their patients about personal and work problems. Additionally, caregivers experienced different kinds of encouragement and support from their patients if their caregiver is feeling stressed and problematic. Patients tend to talk to their caregivers about their problems and that patients give encouraging advice to their health care providers in facing their problems. It is seen to be an effective social support because of the feeling that their patients are mutually responsive to certain conversations about their personal and work related problems. According to a young caregiver,

> *"Our patients tend to make us feel very comfortable when we talk to them about our problems. Even though they are a bit old, they can still comprehend and connect to our present situations."*

The institution is also seen to be a source of social support. Caregivers tend to receive different kinds of help from the institution itself. The institution is seen to be required to help their caregivers in terms of work related problem. Moreover, superiors are expected to encourage caregivers in their work. This is true to some caregivers in the nursing home.

> *"Our superiors taught us everything that we need to do in this nursing home. They serve as our teachers at the same time. They are always there when we need them."*

Having colleagues, family, patients, and other institutional entities as social support is beneficial among caregivers. According to a study by Lau et al. [14], having support from various sources may lead to better wellbeing and good quality of health among individuals. Having different entities as social support systems is beneficial on the part of geriatric palliative caregivers.

3.3.2 Social support function

The function of social support refers to the quality or functional aspects of social support received by caregivers that looks on the roles of their social network provides. The identified social support function received by caregivers are classified into two, intangible support and tangible support (See **Table 5**).

Caregivers receive support that is seen as an encouragement in boosting their psychosocial wellbeing. This refers to the intangible support caregivers receive. This encouragement pertains to the cognitive kind of support that boosts the moral and behavior of caregivers in their personal and work related life. Social support functions as a boosting stimulus to encourage caregivers when feeling depressed or having personal problem. Majority of the caregivers responded that they are

Intangible support	Tangible support
Emotional Support (e.g. talking about problems, boosting self-esteem, etc.)	Monetary support (e.g. lending money, giving incentives)
Informational Support (e.g. sharing knowledge about caregiving)	In-kind support (e.g. sharing food)

Table 5.
Social support function.

mostly encouraged emotionally by the social support they receive. This refers to emotional support. This kind of support indicates that caregivers experience a boost or encouragement on their emotional well-being from different social actors. Conversing with different social actors serves as a way of encouragement for the caregivers to solve their personal and work related problems. According to a female caregiver,

> *"We help each other in this nursing home, if there is someone who needs help; we opt to help them so that they would not get depressed. Even our patients tend to talk to us so that we would not be sad. They would even make us happy. I feel very encouraged when our patients are happy because of our work."*

Information support among caregivers is also cited to be a significant social support function. Different social actors are seen to assist caregivers by giving certain kinds of information most especially to the profession of health care. This kind of social support refers to informational gain support. Most caregivers answered that it is a very important social support they receive. The purpose of informational support is to increase the knowledge of caregivers in tending to their patients. Caregivers admitted that the institution and their colleagues help one another in doing geriatric palliative care to their patients.

> *"We tend to help each other especially if our colleagues need help with their patients. Sometimes, I tend to seek help from them if I do not know what to do. Even our superiors teach us if we do not know what to do."*

Another classification of social support function is tangible support. This refers to the support that can be seen and used by caregivers. This also serves as an encouragement that can be used externally compared to intangible support functions. Most caregivers receive monetary support from different social actors as reinforcement. This is mostly seen by the support given by the institution to the caregivers.

In-kind support also is a kind of tangible support received by caregivers. This refers to food, supplies, and different tangible encouragement given to caregivers. These are mostly given as a sign of appreciation and inspiration from different social actors. This kind of social support is mostly given by the family of patients. According to a female caregiver,

> *"We were given food by the family of our patients because they appreciate that we are caring for their grandparent. They always tell us to take good care of their grandparents."*

All in all, the functions of social support (intangible or tangible) are due to the idea that Filipinos value relationships. According to Medina [22], the function of Filipino social entities such as family and friends as social networks is to provide support to individuals, in this case caregivers, in difficult situations. Caregiving is seen as an exhausting work. The main function of social networks is to help caregivers cope with their current conditions. Caregivers are seen to get through every tiring day with the help of their social networks.

4. Conclusion

In summary, this is a descriptive study of the motivation and social support experiences on geriatric palliative care among 20 purposely chosen geriatric palliative caregivers in Metro Manila. This study looks on the variation of experiences among geriatric palliative caregivers on motivation and social support. The data were analyzed through content analysis by formulating common themes and patterns.

Caregivers cite several of motivations for caregiving. Reasons mentioned are identified to be either intrinsic motivation or extrinsic motivation. Intrinsic motivation being cited are emphatic reasons which include altruistic motivations; emotional reasons such as emotional attachment; and cognitive reasons which refers to gaining knowledge in caregiving. Extrinsic motivations by caregivers are incentive reasons which include monetary gains; and negative reinforcements such as institutional punishments.

In terms of social support received, caregivers mentioned different sources and functions of support they receive. Caregivers cite two types of social support structure or sources, proximal social support and institution based support. For social support function, responses are categorized into intangible and tangible support.

Author details

Wilfred Luis Clamor
De La Salle University, Manila, Philippines

*Address all correspondence to: wilfred.clamor@dlsu.edu.ph

References

[1] Sakakibara, K., Kabayama, M., & Ito, M. (2015). Experiences of "endless" caregiving of impaired elderly at home by family caregivers: a qualitative study. *BMC Research Notes, 8(*827). https://doi.org/10.1186/s13104-015-1829-x

[2] LeSeure, P., & Chongkham-ang, S. (2015). The Experience of Caregivers Living with Cancer Patients: A Systematic Review and Meta-Synthesis. *Journal of Personal. Medicine*, 5, 406—439. doi: 10.3390/ jpm5040406

[3] Pearlin, L., & Schooler, C. (1978). The structure of coping. *Journal of Health and Social Behavior. 19*(1). 2—21. DOI: 10.2307/2136319

[4] Skinner, E. (1996). A guide to constructs of control. [Review]. *Journal of Personality and Social Psychology, 71*(3), 549—570. DOI: 10.1037//0022-3514.71.3.549

[5] Bandura, A. (1986). *Social Foundations of thought and action: A Social cognitive theory.* Prentice Hall

[6] Drentea, P. (2007). Caregiving. In G. Ritzer (Ed.), Blackwell encyclopedia of sociology. [Caregiving]. Blackwell Reference Online. Retrieved http://www.blackwellreference.com/subscriber/book?id=g978140512431_9781405124331

[7] Brown, R., & Brown, M. (2014). Informal caregiving: A reappraisal of effects on caregivers. *Social Issues and Policy Review, 8*, 74—102. https://doi.org/10.1111/sipr.12002

[8] Hyde, P., Harris, C., & Boaden, R. (2013). Pro-social organisational behaviour of health care workers. *International Journal of Human Resource Management, 24*(16), 3115—3130. https://doi.org/10.1080/09585192.2013.775030

[9] Eisenberg, N., & Fabes, R. (1998). Prosocial development. In W. Damon (Series Ed.) and N. Eisenberg (Vol. Ed.), *Handbook of child psychology, 3*, 701—778. https://doi.org/10.1002/9780470147658.chpsy0311

[10] Carlo, G., & Randall, B. A. (2001). Are all prosocial behaviors equal? A socioecological developmental conception of prosocial behavior. In F. Columbus (Ed.), *Advances in psychology research, 2,* 151—170. Nova Science.

[11] Bhatti, K., & Qureshi, T. (2007). Impact of Employee Participation on Job Satisfaction, Employee Commitment and Employee Productivity. *International Review of Business Research Papers, 3*(2), 54—68. https://www.semanticscholar.org/paper/Impact-Of-Employee Participation-On-Job-Employee-Bhatti Qureshi/64f045fcdaca7972323679091047e603790fd269

[12] Benabou, R., & Tirole, J. (2003). Intrinsic and Extrinsic Motivation. *Review of Economic Studies, 70*(3), 489—520. https://doi.org/10.1111/1467-937X.00253

[13] Kreps, D. (1997). Intrinsic Motivation and Extrinsic Incentives. *American Economic Review, 87*(2), 359—364. https://www.jstor.org/stable/2950946

[14] Lau, D., Berman, R., Halpern, L., Pickard, S., Schrauf. R., & Witt, W. (2010). Exploring Factors that Influence Informal Caregiving in Medication Management for Home Hospice Patients. *Journal of Palliative Medicine, 13*(9), 1085—1090. DOI: 10.1089/jpm.2010.0082

[15] Albrecht, T., & Adelman, M. (1987). Communicating social support: A theoretical perspective. T. Albrecht & M. Adelman (Eds.), *Communicating social support*, 18—39. Sage.

[16] Taylor, S. (2011). Social support: A Review. In M.S. Friedman. *The Handbook of Health Psychology*. Oxford University Press. 189-214.

[17] Wills, T. (1991). Social support and interpersonal relationships. *Prosocial Behavior, Review of Personality and Social Psychology*, 12, 265-289.

[18] Broadhead, W., Gehlbach, S., deGruy, F., & Kaplan, B. (1989). Functional versus structural social support and health care utilization in a family medicine outpatient practice, *Medical Care, 27*(3), 221-233. doi: 10.1097/00005650-198903000-00001.

[19] Langford, C., Bowsher, J., Maloney, J., Lillis, P. (1997). Social support: a conceptual analysis. *Journal of Advanced Nursing. 25,* 95-100. DOI: 10.1046/j.1365-2648.1997.1997025095.x

[20] Kaufman, A., Kosberg, J., Leeper, J., & Tang, M. (2010). Social support, caregiver burden, and life satisfaction in a sample of rural african American and white caregivers of older persons with Dementia. *Journal of Gerontological Social Work, 53,* 251-269. DOI: 10.1080/01634370903478989

[21] Rogers, N. (1999). Caring for those who care. *Adaptation & Aging, 24*(1), 1-12. https://doi.org/10.1300/J016v24n01_01

[22] Medina, B. (2001) *The Filipino Family*. 2nd edition. University of the Philippines Press

[23] Morillo, H., Capuno, J., & Mendoza, A. (2013). Views and values on family among Filipinos: An empirical exploration. *Asian Journal of Social Science, 41*(1), 5—28. https://doi.org/10.1163/15685314-12341278

[24] Cicirelli, V. (1993). Attachment and obligation as daughters' motives for caregiving behavior and subsequent effect on subjective burden. *Psychology and Aging, 8*(2), 144-155. DOI: 10.1037//0882-7974.8.2.144

Chapter 12

The Influence of *Candida* spp. in Intestinal Microbiota; Diet Therapy, the Emerging Conditions Related to *Candida* in Athletes and Elderly People

Alexandru Vasile Rusu, Berta Alvarez Penedo, Ann-Kristin Schwarze and Monica Trif

Abstract

The presence of *Candida* in the gut is normal, but an overproduction may lead to serious health problems due to an imbalanced gut, causing gut-related symptoms such as bowel movement changes, excessive gas, etc. Some diseases, such as Crohn's disease and ulcerative colitis, are associated with an overgrowth of *Candida* in the gastrointestinal tract. Several recent studies have shown that a prolonged candidiasis within the intestines is associated with *Candida* overgrowth syndrome or chronic fatigue syndrome. A healthy digestive system relies on a good balance of bacteria that live in the gut, and an important role in maintaining this balance is having the ingested type of food. *Candida* overgrowth can be prevented first of all by healthy eating patterns, as susceptibility is increased by a high-sugar diet and diabetes or nutritional deficiencies causing a dysregulated immune system. In general, *Candida*-associated conditions have a high impact on performance. Recent research has shown an increasing interest in the *Candida*-related conditions and diseases.

Keywords: physiology, gastrointestinal conditions, gut microbiota, elderly, athletes, diet therapy

1. Introduction

Everyone has yeasts like *Candida* spp., mostly Candida albicans, in their intestines, and only seriously ill people will get sick. In contrast, other therapists fear life-threatening diseases if these germs are detected [1].

Many patients are completely unsettled. These are very seriously ill patients such as cancer or AIDS patients whose defense is extremely weakened [2]. In their cases, the internal organs can fail due to a fungal attack. Fungal diseases and intestinal mycoses have actually increased in recent years. Gynecologists observe that more and more women suffer from vaginal mycoses.

The reasons for this increase are, for example, nutritional errors such as too much sugar and white flour products or nutritional deficiencies causing a dysregulated immune system [3]. However, treatments with cortisone and antibiotics and the increase in environmental pollutants are also contributing factors. All of these factors weaken our immune system and thus promote the spread of the fungi. If, for example, antibiotics have damaged the natural intestinal flora, *Candida* yeasts can spread because important physiological germs are lacking as opponents.

Unfortunately there are only nonspecific symptoms that can have many other causes. In the foreground are diarrhea and constipation—often alternating—flatulence, an abdominal distension, and abdominal pain. Affected people reported migraines, depression, liver diseases, and skin changes. But symptoms may or may not be due to *Candida*.

When referring to the intestinal yeasts, it is usually of *Candida* genus. Yeasts can be found practically everywhere in nature: they colonize the mucous membranes of humans and animals, adhere to objects, and can be found in water and soil. *C. albicans* are commonly found in the intestine. These yeasts were previously found in 80% of all intestinal yeast infections. In contrast to other *Candida* species, *C. albicans* adheres to the mucous membranes of warm-blooded humans and animals. Their transmission takes place directly through physical contact. In healthy people, however, this is completely unproblematic. But there are also numerous other types of *Candida* that have been on the rise recently. Yeasts find optimal living conditions in the intestine as the environment meets their requirements and provides them plenty of food [4].

People with weakened immune systems are particularly at risk of contracting *Candida*. Older people (elderly), whose defenses are weakening, are also considered a high-risk group [5].

The role of intestinal gut microbiota in health and disease is gaining more attention and is increasingly recognized [6]. The philosophy of alimentation might give us a clear start to see the patient as a whole again. It cannot only be drugs and medicine to treat the diseases [7].

2. *Candida* spp. as member of the human gastrointestinal tract microbiota

In the normal human gastrointestinal tract microbiota, *Candida* species are part of and can be found in the oropharynx, esophagus, gastrointestinal tract, and vagina. When the immune system is compromised from different reasons, a local or invasive infection can be developed [5, 8].

Candida species are among the most common yeast, and as fungi in stool cultures, the most common germ is *C. albicans*. *C. albicans* is one of the optionally pathogenic fungi that only trigger a disease under certain conditions [1, 9, 10]. However, numerous other types of fungi can also be detected in healthy intestinal flora in small numbers of germs using modern methods. With reduced immune defense like with HIV disease, but also with diabetes mellitus or cancer and with therapies with immune inhibitors (immunosuppressive therapy, e.g., with steroids [cortisone]), the amount of *Candida* in the intestine can increase significantly, so that a serious disease becomes possible [2].

Overgrowth of the intestine (over 1,000,000 fungi/g stool) is often accompanied by annoying gas, intestinal cramps, and/or diarrhea. If such symptoms occur in patients with a weakened immune system, overgrowth with *Candida* should also be considered [11–13].

3. *Candida* hypersensitivity syndrome

Candida hypersensitivity syndrome was first described 20 years ago. For many years, *C. albicans* has been mentioned as the cause of *Candida* hypersensitivity syndrome. This chronic syndrome is also known as chronic candidiasis, *Candida*-related complex, and "the yeast connection" [14].

A *Candida* "infection" or colonization—not proven—is associated with a variety of diseases, e.g., cancer, permanent fatigue and exhaustion, depression, and headache. In addition, there is always speculation that the irritable bowel may have to do with an overgrowth of fungi in the intestine. Still enough scientific evidence is lacking [15–17].

Candida is often held responsible for unspecific physical complaints or symptoms. As explained above, the simple detection of fungi in the intestinal flora in small numbers does not justify the start of a corresponding therapy [18]. Extensive and often costly treatment methods such as stool enema, colonic hydrotherapy, detoxification, and antifungal diets are particularly special or rejecting self-urine therapy as unscientific and unsuccessful [19].

Symptoms such as fatigue general malaise and genitourinary and neuropsychiatric complaints and nonspecific gastrointestinal symptoms are reported.

The syndrome is considered to be caused by vaginal and intestinal fungal overgrowth, production of fungal toxins, inflammation, and invasion of mucous membranes. In such conditions, the usual therapy will consist of a rigorous long-term antifungal treatment and "yeast elimination" diet [20–22].

A nutritional imbalance demonstrated by diet analysis could lead to the development of further nutritional deficiencies for a prolonged period of time diet [19, 23].

4. An overview of *Candida*-related conditions in athletes' case: impact on athlete physiological performance capacity

Exercise has a strong impact in an athlete's body. In fact, intense exercise, and particularly endurance exercise, requires an adaptive regulation of athletes' body in order to fulfill the new physiological and biochemical demands. Under these stimuli, the muscle adapts by improving its metabolic, mechanical, contractile, and neuromuscular functions [24]. Glycogen storage decreases, mitochondrial biogenesis increases, and the balance of electrolytes varies [25]. Moreover, in response to the higher demand of oxygen and nutrients by the muscle, cardiac output, ventilation, and gas exchange increase, which finally results in an increased vascular dilatation. Exercise increases the risk of dehydration as a result of the increment of body temperature. In order to compensate for and reestablish the homeostatic equilibrium, the amount of glucocorticoids and adrenaline release should be higher [26, 27]. Furthermore, blood flow decreases in the liver, pancreas, and kidneys where metabolism activity increases.

Exercise also damages the muscle and highly influences systemic inflammation, intestinal permeability, and an increase in oxidative stress as well as immune response, all of them being related with delayed onset muscle soreness (DOMS) [28].

DOMS is a muscle pain or discomfort that begins after unaccustomed or high-intensity exercise [29]. Usually the peak of the pain appears 1–3 days after exercise and can last for 5–7 days postexercise [30]. DOMS is recognized as one of the most frequent and recurrent forms of sport injury affecting both athletic (including elite athletes) and nonathletic population. Its prevalence is higher when exercise activity increases (e.g., beginning of sporting season) or when a new type of activity is introduced. Duration and intensity of exercise also influence DOMS. Thereby, intense exercise is related to higher degrees of DOMS, immune system suppression, inflammation, and oxidative stress, while low-to-moderate exercise is related with enhancing the immune system and healthy lifestyle. Despite its high incidence, the mechanisms of DOMS remain uncertain, and there are no specific treatment strategies. DOMS can negatively affect several factors of athletic performance such as muscular pain, reduced joint range of motion, power reduction, altered muscle sequencing and recruitment patterns, and muscular strength [29]. Additionally, DOMS affects athletic performance by increasing the risk of other muscle injuries but also by making athletes more prone to suffer from opportunistic infections such as candidiasis. This may be mainly because of the underlying state of chronic inflammation due to exercise, altered immune system, and oxidative stress. Actually, infectious diseases and particularly fungal infections [31] have been identified as the most common and important health problems in athletes [32], especially in contact sports. Some studies found that among wrestlers, skin infections are a common cause of training and match disruption, thus directly affecting athletic performance [31]. Also it has been determined that *C. albicans*, one of the most important causative agents of opportunistic infections, was responsible of those infections in 5% of the analyzed athletic population [9]. Therefore, it can be assumed that the alterations due to the impact of exercise (mainly increase of inflammation, affected immune system, and oxidative stress) may alter gut microbiota, increasing the risk of opportunistic infections such as *Candida* infections. Other studies found that in comparison with controls, athletes used twice as frequently oral antibiotics [33]. This supports the hypothesis that specific variations in gut microbiota may even be the starting point of different diseases development [34].

Diet and nutritional or dietary supplements have been identified as the main factor affecting gut microbiota (**Table 1**). In fact, it has been proven that dietetic changes can induce up to 57% of gut microbiota [35] variations in terms of composition and functioning in 24 hours [36, 37]. On the other hand, several studies have demonstrated the influence that gut microbiota have on essential processes affecting the individual's health and performance (e.g., immune response and metabolism of nutrients) [34, 38]. Therefore, it could be assumed that diet and food supplements (also called nutritional or dietary supplements) may be a critical factor through which gut microbiota can be modulated in order to benefit athletes in their performance. Actually a recent study has identified several dietetic patterns which address this idea [39].

Most studies analyzing the impact of probiotics in athletic performance highlight their positive impact on the immune function, gut mucosa permeability, and oxidative stress resulting from intense exercise but also they increase the risk of respiratory diseases that are very common in athletes [40]. Thus, probiotics have been proven to improve athletes' performance.

Up to now, there is no specific information on how diet and food supplements directly affect *Candida* and how *Candida* further impact athletic performance. However, interesting data shown may give a hint regarding *Candida* behavior with respect to probiotic consumption [41]. A study [41] evaluated healthy young individuals and analyzed the impact that probiotics consumption has on the presence of *Candida* in oral cavity. Results show 46% reduction in *Candida* prevalence after probiotics consumption in oral cavity. *C. albicans* was the main *Candida* spp. identified followed by *C. tropicalis* [42].

Finally, evidence supports that also antibiotics influence gut microbiota composition. The use of antibiotics increases the risk of opportunistic candidiasis

Nutrient	Dose	Effect
Carbohydrates	7–12 g/kg/day (endurance athletes)	A fatigue reduction and an improved performance and mood can be achieved during an intense training by consuming high doses of carbohydrates ad libitum
Proteins	1.2–1.6 g/kg/day (elite athletes)	The infection incidents increase due to a protein deficiency by decreasing the T cell functions which affect the immunity system
Fat	15–30% of the diet/day	A reduction of the intestinal inflammation, bacterial translocation, and gastrointestinal stress can be achieved by fat diets with good amount of omega-3 and omega-6 However, a high-fat diet may reduce the total gut microbiota
Fiber	38 g/day man 25 g/day women	Lower level gut microbiota is associated with low-fiber diet and low antipathogenic bacteria and therefore will be an increase in gut inflammation and less sympathetic nervous system stimulation However, gastrointestinal stress may be caused by a high-fiber diet
Probiotics	Highly variable depending on the strain, microbial composition, and metagenome Because of gut microbiota diversity in humans, there was not established a standard dose	Supplementing the diet with fermented food can stimulate the expansion of microorganism like *Bifidobacteria* (*B.*) and *Lactobacillus* (*L.*) that have beneficial metabolic functions. For example, improving short-chain fatty acids results in an increasing immune and barrier functions

Table 1.
Dietary modifications for the improvement of gut microbiota [39].

infections. Additionally, it has been also reported that antibiotics may cause fatigue and therefore negatively influence athletic performance [41]. Research done to analyze the relation between the total use of antibiotics (duration of antibiotic courses) and the degree of fatigue has shown that the longer the antibiotic courses, the higher the fatigue scores obtained [43, 44].

Lately studies evaluated the ergogenic effect of probiotic supplementation and their effect on physical exercises, trying to identify their mechanisms of action and on how could they influence the improvement of performance. Due to the fact that only few studies were performed and demonstrated the ergogenic effect of probiotics, further studies should investigate the subject for better understanding [45–52].

5. An overview of *Candida*-related conditions in elderly case: physiological alterations

The term "elderly" comprises those individuals aged 60 and older, and they represent the fastest growing population group. In fact, in 2017 the global population of 60 years old and over totaled 962 million, and it is foreseen to reach 2.1 billion by 2050 [53]. Already by 2030 it is anticipated that nearly 35% of the European population will be over 60 and 11% over 80 years [53]. With age progression, deficiencies of physiological functions occur, making elderly more vulnerable to diseases and infections, particularly from fungal species [54]. Genus *Candida* is considered the most important cause of opportunistic infections affecting especially immunocompromised patients and elderly people and the major causative agent of nosocomial infections [55]. The step from *Candida* colonization to subsequent infection is not yet clear. However it has been proven that the natural flora which develops within the gastrointestinal tract can represent the main source in the development of severe infections.

Candida infections are very difficult to diagnose in the elderly and have a complicated therapeutic management [56]. Signs and symptoms are often nonspecific and can vary depending on the area affected. Thus, diagnosis depends on the clinical evaluation supported by biochemical and microbiological analysis. Given the difficulty of diagnosing *Candida* infection, efforts have been focused on the development of new strategies and diagnosis methods such as new culture methods with increased sensitivity. Also novel antigen-based tests are available for the detection of mannan levels which is the main component of *Candida* cell wall and 1,3-β-D-glucan which is mainly used in critically ill patients as it has high sensitivity [54, 57]. Finally, real-time polymerase chain reaction technique is also applied for the detection of five different *Candida* spp. [54].

Regarding the epidemiology, 90% of all *Candida* infections are caused by *C. krusei*, *C. glabrata*, *C. albicans*, *C. tropicalis*, and *C. parapsilosis* [58].

Aging-related physiological changes and other factors frequently affecting the elderly such as comorbidities, polypharmacy, and high colonization rate result in an extremely high mortality rate (from 36 to 63%) [59].

The oral cavity is considered a major physiological importance and experiences numerous alterations with aging process. The impaired functioning of the salivary gland alters the quality and quantity of saliva (hyposalivation). This impacts the equilibrium of the resident oral microbiota and also results in the decrease of defensive proteins (such as salivary peroxidases or myeloperoxidase) as well as other substances with antimicrobial activity (e.g., lysozymes), facilitating the development of oral candidiasis. Using removable dental prostheses and their deficient hygienization also contribute to oral candidiasis. *C. albicans* followed by *C. glabrata* and *C. tropicalis* have been identified as the most prevalent *Candida* spp. found in dental prostheses [60]. The use of drugs that irritate or damage the oral mucosa, such as long-term antibiotic intake, as well as the presence of chronic and/or concurrent diseases may also lead to candidiasis. As already mentioned, *Candida* colonization can lead to severe infections. Thus, from oral cavity colonization, *Candida* may increase the colonization index and reach easier other areas such as the respiratory system [61].

Further, oral candidiasis may lead to appetite decline, and this can limit the nutrient intake which can directly influence gut microbiota growth. Appetite decline can also be a consequence of other age-related physiological alterations (**Table 2**) [62]. The impaired masticatory efficiency produced by poor dental health and related pain, loss of teeth and muscle bulk, and lower sensitivity (including taste, smell, and sight) have a negative influence on appetite as food remains uninteresting [62, 63]. Oropharyngeal and esophageal motility diminished the risk of swallowing impairments (e.g., dysphagia) and prevalence of gastroesophageal reflux. Additionally, alterations in the secretion and peripheral action of the hormones that regulate the wish to eat, hunger, and satiation can also reduce appetite. Besides the reduction of appetite, the nutritional status of the elderly can be influenced by the changes in gastrointestinal motility which can lead to reduced digestion and absorption, among others. All those result in the changes in the availability of nutrients in the gut which influence the abundance of *Candida* and may lead to dysbiosis. For example, it has been proven that a high-fat diet stimulated the increase in Firmicutes and Proteobacteria and a decrease in Bacteroidetes [64]. Poor nutrition has been also proven to be associated with the development of inflammatory pathologies (e.g. Crohn's disease) and chronic disease associated with

Natural aging physiological alterations
Alterations in oral cavity (e.g. hyposalivation and impaired masticatory efficiency)
Alterations in the secretion and peripheral action of the hormones that regulate the wish to eat, hunger, and satiation
Changes in gastrointestinal motility
Immunosenescence (alterations in immune system such as decreased phagocytosis and age-related involution of the thymus or altersinvolution)
Changes in gut microbiota
Altered metabolism of certain drugs
Decreased renal function
Decreased hepatic function

Table 2.
Natural aging physiological alterations.

nutritional status (e.g., diabetes mellitus and cardiovascular diseases). Finally, poor nutrition can also derive in malnutrition which is one of the key factors influencing the growth of gut microbiota and, thus, may also lead to the dysregulation of the immune system and posterior infection.

The immune system is also affected with aging (a process known as immunosenescence) [65]. Hence, there have been identified several altered immune parameters as well as adaptive and innate immunity influencing the development of chronic inflammatory status. Also the composition of gut microbiota varies with aging [66]. It decreases the number and variety of many protective commensal anaerobes such as lactobacilli and bifidobacteria. Beside this, phagocytosis is altered as a consequence of the functional insufficiency of monocytes and macrophages. On the other hand, "altersinvolution" (referring to age-related involution of the thymus) leads in a decline in circulating antigen-presenting cells (e.g., dendritic and T cells) [67]; T cells show altered cytokine production and lose their memory capacity as well as decrease the number of circulating B cells. Consequently, the immune system is compromised, and thus, there is a higher risk for the elderly to develop serious fungal infections, especially disseminated candidiasis. The source of this infection is often the gastrointestinal tract. The administration of broad-spectrum antimicrobial agents to these patients increases their risk of *Candida* infections by increasing the frequency and magnitude of gastrointestinal tract colonization by *Candida* spp.

Physiological changes associated with aging also affect the metabolism of many drugs [68]. As time passes, the hepatic capacity diminishes, affecting drug clearance. Specifically, the microsomal cytochrome P450-dependent monooxygenase system is altered, and therefore, the drugs that undergo this pathway cannot be cleaned properly. Liver volume and blood flow also decline, impacting drug clearance. In addition renal size and volume are reduced. There are less glomeruli and juxtamedullary nephrons, resulting in a decrease in filtration area of the glomerular basement membrane and decreased permeability. Thus, the glomerular filtration rate (GFR) is decreased [69]. Both liver and renal modifications impact the elderly's pharmacokinetics and pharmacodynamics variables, thus making them at higher risk of adverse drug reactions and harmful drug interactions. Together with the above information, other common factors such as serious underlying diseases and comorbidities, the use of antibiotics and immunosuppressive drugs, living in care facilities, or being hospitalized increase the risk of the elderly suffering from *Candida*-induced infections (particularly *Candida* oral infections) and make them more vulnerable.

For frail elderly, severe surgeries, the use of central venous catheter, and parenteral nutrition are associated with candidemia related to biofilm formation and hence persistent colonization and infections [70]. Biofilm formation by an irreversible adhesion of a community of microorganisms which attached to each other on a surface, inert material, or living tissue, produce extracellular polymers that provide a structural matrix. The microorganism in this community behaves differently, showing more resistance to antibiotics and lower growth rates. Different *Candida* spp. have been identified to be implicated in biofilm formation. Each of them exhibits particularities in terms of biofilm formations (morphology, extracellular matrix, antifungal resistance, etc.) and thus complicating treatment. *C. parapsilosis* has been characterized as the most frequently causative agent of catheter-related infections through biofilm formation [71]. It is an exogenous pathogen found mostly on the skin of healthy hosts which easily spread through hand contamination in hospitals and care facilities. *C. tropicalis* is particularly relevant in urinary tract infections [72, 73].

6. *Candida* elimination diet therapy

An important point is the amount of fungi found in the intestine. Antibiotic treatments are damaging the natural intestinal flora, and fungi such as *Candida* spread because important physiological germs are lacking as opponents [74]. Treatments such as antibody therapies or enteral nutrition can reduce the inflammation, and gut microbiota is improved.

A dietary formula for 1 week lacking fiber reduced the populations of fungi [75]. Therefore, it is believed that the gastrointestinal environment can be restored by a proper defined nutrition diet formula [76–78].

Such diets are high in sugar and total carbohydrates which are correlated with increased methanogen *Methanobrevibacter* and fungus *Candida* and other genera from different domains of life that are negatively associated with the consumption of fatty acids, protein, and amino acids [79].

Candida is the predominant fungal species capable of colonizing the gut and can vary extensively in time in response to recent carbohydrate consumption, antibiotic use, and environmental sources. Bacterial population structure primarily associates with long-term diet [80]. In a recent study, *Candida* correlated positively with long-term intake of total carbohydrates and sugar and had a strong association with recent carbohydrate intake.

Short-chain fatty acids (SCFAs) have been shown to exert fungistatic effect. Anaerobic intestinal microbiota, such as lactic acid bacteria (LAB) as a member of normal flora, produces from dietary fibers via fermentation of beneficial metabolites, and the major end products are SCFAs. Not only for the intestinal microbiota, SCFAs represent an energy substrate but for host cells as well. Their important role in reducing the development of gastrointestinal disorders, among others, is well-known, preventing overgrowth of *Candida* [81].

The probiotic strain *L. rhamnosus* GG offers benefit human health, and is a commonly used probiotic strain with immunomodulatory effect and bears an exopolysaccharide interfering with *Candida* growth and invasion tested in a model of gastrointestinal candidiasis, mostly attributed to *C. albicans* [82]. SCFAs have an effect on morphogenesis and therefore may provide a mechanism by which LAB could prevent candidal colonization. The growth rates are crucial for fungal growth in medium containing the disaccharide maltose as a sole nutrient source [74, 81].

In a clinical study performed in individuals with chronic intestinal *Candida* overgrowth receiving nystatin alone and following a diet therapy (avoiding foods high in simple sugars and starch), different cured rates have been achieved during the 3 months of tests, 42% compared to 85% [21].

The yeasts metabolize a part of the carbohydrates from food, producing carbon dioxide and fusel alcohols. The gas causes an abdominal distension, bloating, and abdominal pain. Prolonged exposure to fusel alcohols for weeks and months can damage the liver. It was only this spring that a special toxin produced by the *Candida* yeast was found, which is responsible for many of the effects on other parts of the body. There is still a lot of research to be done in this area.

Most of the usual antifungal diets are based on the elimination of sugar and other carbohydrates and can actually relieve bloating and other irritable bowel symptoms in some patients (with or without fungal overgrowth) [83, 84]. Practitioners of alternative medicine often claim that candidiasis—the most common cause of yeast infections (vaginal candidiasis) and oral thrush (oral candidiasis)—can be treated or prevented with diet and food supplements [11]. Despite a lack of clinical evidence, *Candida* diets have become incredibly popular in recent years, mostly among women with recurrent yeast infections.

The effect is probably based on a combination of different changes at the level of bacterial flora, the formation and transport mechanisms of intestinal gas, and the osmotic properties of the intestinal contents. The concept of the *Candida* diet is that *Candida* uses sugar compounds (carbohydrates) to extract energy from them. If these sugar compounds are no longer available through the diet, the *Candida* can be "starved" in this way [85].

The *Candida* yeasts break down carbohydrates from food into carbon dioxide and fusel alcohols. The gas causes a bloated stomach, a feeling of fullness, and pain in the intestinal area. If the exposure to fusel alcohols lasts longer, they can damage the liver. The *Candida* yeast produces a special toxin that has only recently been identified and can trigger symptoms such as migraines or joint illnesses [86].

A consistent antifungal diet of at least 5–6 weeks is also essential. It is important to deprive the yeast of their base food. Sugar, sweets, white flour products, and alcohol should be strictly avoided. Sweet fruit should also be avoided in the first 4 weeks. The focus is on a wholesome diet with lots of lettuce, vegetables, and whole grain products. The high-fiber diet not only strengthens the immune system but also presumably exerts a mechanical cleaning effect by sweeping the fungal nests out of the villi through its fibrous structure and at the same time stimulating the bowel movement [87, 88]. High-content phytochemicals with an antimicrobial effect make the whole-food diet the ideal antifungal diet—however, success is only permanent if there is a consequent change in diet.

Whole foods are the best way to prevent yeast infections. The yeasts will not find the right breeding ground in the organism of a healthy person. If there is already an infection, targeted therapy and a long-term change in eating habits to a healthy, natural diet are effective remedies.

In microbiological therapy, the focus is on strengthening the immune system [89]. Bacteria are extremely important for an intact immune system. An estimated 100 trillion bacteria live in the intestine, many of which are not yet known. It is now known that these bacteria have important functions for the immune system and are not simply there by accident. Experience after lengthy antibiotic administration speaks about, again and again, weaknesses in the body's defenses which are observed because these active ingredients not only destroy unwanted but also desired bacteria. In our environment, which is enlivened by countless germs, the animals die of fatal infections after a few days because their defense system is practically inadequate. The contact with bacteria is very important for the development of the immune system. This effect is mimicked with microbiological therapy. The patients are given probiotics and auto-vaccines for 3–6 months. Probiotics are preparations from intestinal germs that regulate the immune system. Several studies suggested that certain *Lactobacillus* probiotic strains enhance the effect of antifungal drugs (like fluconazole) used to treat yeast infections. However, there was no evidence that the strains could achieve the same effect on their own [90–95].

The use of probiotics in treating yeast infections is controversial. Although probiotics work by increasing bacteria beneficial to the vagina and gastrointestinal tract, their ability to prevent or treat candidiasis is a subject to debate. While many studies suggest that a daily probiotic can "slightly improve" imbalances that lead to yeast infections, others do not [96].

With these foods too, some of the bacteria will certainly live in the intestine. It is probably not possible to permanently colonize these bacteria in the intestine. However, a distinction must be made between probiotic medication and food. Special foods, such as yogurt preparations, cannot be used to inject as many bacteria as with medication. Patients would have to eat tons of yogurts in order to achieve a therapeutically effective number of bacteria. Then, however, they would have problems with the masses of animal protein again.

To permanently eliminate the yeast, a change in eating habits is crucial. The yeast must be deprived of their food base. It is very important to avoid sugar. In the acute diet phase of 4 weeks, patients even have to do without sweet fruits because *Candida* can also utilize fructose. Only sour apples, lemons, and grapefruit are allowed. The focus is on a high-fiber diet, which means a lot of salad and vegetables as well as whole grains [97, 98]. Their fiber exerts a mechanical "cleaning effect" by sweeping out the fungal nests between the villi, and they stimulate the movement of the intestine. In addition, fiber is cheap because it cannot be broken down by the yeast in the intestine. We therefore recommend our patients to eat whole foods.

The complex carbohydrates and especially the fiber are digested in the lower intestinal sections. However, the yeasts mainly colonize the upper sections because they require oxygen. Only relatively few yeasts can survive in the colon. Only an insignificant part of the yeast uses the complex carbohydrates and fiber [99].

The die-off effects (*Candida* dies) can be strong, especially at the beginning of treatment when a large amount of *Candida* fungi dies at once. Likely massive adrenal fatigue can be experienced during this period. In this case, the recommendation is to take a couple of weeks off not to add any new foods to diet. Die-off is usually a problem from the beginning to about the middle of treatment. As healing progresses, the die-off symptoms (like the other *Candida* symptoms) will occur less frequently and at greater intervals. Therefore, at the same time with the diet, it is highly recommended to start with antifungals and probiotics. The combination of these two kills the *Candida* yeast in the intestine and immediately populates it with "good bacteria."

An antifungal diet always represents an individual nutritional concept, which in general is based on the results of laboratory analysis. In the case of a stronger fungal attack, an antifungal medication is recommended. The microbiological therapy is often useful, since the intestinal flora is usually affected; otherwise the fungi would not have been able to multiply.

Candidiasis affecting the whole organism is fatal in about 70% of cases. The problem is *Candida*-induced sepsis, in which the pathogens can be found in large numbers in the blood. Around 40,000 people in Germany are affected by this invasive *Candida* infection every year. When it comes to hospital infections, it represents number 4 on the list of the most dangerous pathogens [100].

7. Conclusions

Numerous microorganisms live in our intestines, especially *Candida*. As long as the intestinal flora is in natural balance, *Candida* does not cause problems.

In people whose immune systems are weakened by disease or medication—the elderly population, *C. albicans* can also cause inflammation. The problem is that a *Candida* infection is often diagnosed late because of its diverse symptoms.

The *Candida* diet is believed to limit *Candida* colonization and thus prevent such opportunistic infections. The *Candida* diet's aim and scope are boosting the immunity, reducing inflammation, and improving gut health. The diet is based on removing added sugars, focusing on consumption of fermented foods, and avoiding pro-inflammatory triggers. By providing an optimal nutrition, a reduction of inflammation and depriving *C. albicans* will be possible. Antifungal diet is believed to greatly reduce the number of microorganisms in the intestine within at least 4 weeks.

Nevertheless, it is recommended to carry out the diet under medical supervision, especially if there are problems with the intestinal flora.

Acknowledgements

This work has received funding from the European Union's Horizon 2020 research and innovation program under grant agreement No. 816303 (STANCE4HEALTH).

Conflict of interest

The authors declare no conflict of interest.

Author details

Alexandru Vasile Rusu[1*], Berta Alvarez Penedo[1], Ann-Kristin Schwarze[1] and Monica Trif[2*]

1 Biozoon Food Innovations GmbH, Bremerhaven, Germany

2 Centre for Innovative Process Engineering GmbH, Stuhr, Germany

*Address all correspondence to: rusu@biozoon.de and monica_trif@hotmail.com

References

[1] Kim J, Sudbery P. *Candida albicans*, a major human fungal pathogen. Journal of Microbiology. 2011;**49**(2):171-177

[2] Brennan CA, Garrett WS. Gut microbiota, inflammation, and colorectal cancer. Annual Review of Microbiology. 2016;**70**:395-411

[3] Conlon MA, Bird AR. The impact of diet and lifestyle on gut microbiota and human health. Nutrients. 2015;**7**:17-44

[4] Tomasello G, Mazzola M, Jurjus A, et al. The fingerprint of the human gastrointestinal tract microbiota: A hypothesis of molecular mapping. Journal of Biological Regulators and Homeostatic Agents. 2017;**31**(1):245-249

[5] Dekkers BGJ, Veringa A, Marriott DJE, Boonstra JM, van der Elst KCM, Doukas FF, et al. Invasive candidiasis in the elderly: Considerations for drug therapy. Drugs & Aging. 2018;**35**:781-789

[6] Hallen-Adams HE, Suhr MJ. Fungi in the healthy human gastrointestinal tract. Virulence. 2017;**8**(3):352-358

[7] Meral G. Philosophy of Nutrition: Past-Future Nutrition, Gut Microbiota - Brain Axis, Alper Evrensel and Barış Önen Ünsalver. Rijeka: IntechOpen; 2018

[8] Ignatova V. Influence of gut microbiota on behavior and its disturbances. In: Palermo S, Morese R, editors. Behavioral Neuroscience. Rijeka: IntechOpen; 2019

[9] Yapar N. Epidemiology and risk factors for invasive candidiasis. Therapeutics and Clinical Risk Management. 2014;**10**:95-105

[10] Kosmidis C, Denning DW. Chapter 189—Opportunistic and systemic fungi. In: Cohen J, Opal SM, William G, editors. Infectious Diseases. 4th Edition. Elsevier. Vol. 2. 2017. pp. 1681-1709.e3. Available from: https://doi.org/10.1016/B978-0-7020-6285-8.00189-1

[11] Richardson JP, Moyes DL. Adaptive immune responses to *Candida albicans* infection. Virulence. 2015;**6**(4):327-337

[12] Höfs S, Mogavero S, Hube B. Interaction of *Candida albicans* with host cells: Virulence factors, host defense, escape strategies, and the microbiota. Journal of Microbiology. 2016;**54**:149-169

[13] Limon JJ, Skalski JH, Underhill DM. Commensal fungi in health and disease. Cell Host & Microbe. 2017;**22**(2):156-165

[14] Marshall GS, Carter BD. Chronic fatigue syndrome. In: Long SS, editor. Principles and Practice of Pediatric Infectious Diseases. New York. 2018. pp. 1037-1044.e6. In press

[15] Clapp M, Aurora N, Herrera L, Bhatia M, Wilen E, Wakefield S. Gut microbiota's effect on mental health: The gut-brain axis. Clinical Practice. 2017;**7**(4):987

[16] Fuertes A, Pérez-Burillo S, Apaolaza I, Vallès Y, Francino MP, Rufián-Henares JÁ, et al. Adaptation of the human gut microbiota metabolic network during the first year after birth. Frontiers in Microbiology. 2019;**10**:848

[17] Zanoaga O, Braicu C, Jurj A, Rusu A, Buiga R, Berindan-Neagoe I. Progress in research on the role of flavonoids in lung Cancer. International Journal of Molecular Sciences. 2019;**20**(17):4291

[18] Nocerino A, Nguyen A, Agrawal M, Mone A, Lakhani K, Swaminath A. Fatigue in inflammatory bowel diseases:

Etiologies and management. Advances in Therapy. 2020;**37**(1):97-112

[19] Singh RK, Chang HW, Yan D, Lee KM, Ucmak D, Wong K, et al. Influence of diet on the gut microbiome and implications for human health. Journal of Translational Medicine. 2017;**15**(1):73

[20] Valdes AM, Walter J, Segal E, Spector TD. Role of the gut microbiota in nutrition and health. BMJ. 2018;**361**:k2179

[21] Otasevic S, Momcilovic S, Petrovic M, Radulovic O, Stojanovic NM, Arsic-Arsenijevic V. The dietary modification and treatment of intestinal *Candida* overgrowth—A pilot study. Journal de Mycologie Medicale. 2018;**28**:623-627

[22] Leeming ER, Johnson AJ, Spector TD, Le Roy CI. Effect of diet on the gut microbiota: Rethinking intervention duration. Nutrients. 2019;**11**:2862

[23] Forstner S. Rusu a. Development of Personalised Food for the Nutrition of Elderly Consumers. Know your Food: Food Ethics and Innovation. Wageningen: Wageningen Academic Publishers; 2015. pp. S. 24-S. 27

[24] Russell AP, Lamon S, Boon H, Wada S, Güller I, Brown AVC, et al. Regulation of miRNAs in human skeletal muscle following acute endurance exercise and short-term endurance training. The Journal of Physiology. 2013;**591**(Pt 18):4637-4653

[25] Munoz A, Riber C, Trigo C, Castejón-Riber C, Castejón FM. Dehydration, electrolyte imbalances and renin-angiotensin-aldosterone-vasopressin axis in successful and unsuccessful endurance horses. Equine Veterinary Journal. Supplement. 2010;**42**:83-90

[26] Sharara-Chami RI, Joachim M, Pacak K, Majzoub JA. Glucocorticoid treatment—effect on adrenal medullary catecholamine production. Shock. 2010;**33**(2):213-217

[27] Nicolaides NC, Pavlaki AN, Maria Alexandra MA, et al. Glucocorticoid therapy and adrenal suppression. In: Feingold KR, Anawalt B, Boyce A, et al., editors. Endotext [Internet]. South Dartmouth (MA): MDText.com, Inc.; 2000. [Updated 2018 Oct 19]

[28] Fernández-Lázaro D, Mielgo-Ayuso J, Seco Calvo J, Córdova Martínez A, Caballero García A, Fernandez-Lazaro CI. Modulation of exercise-induced muscle damage, inflammation, and oxidative markers by curcumin supplementation in a physically active population: A systematic review. Nutrients. 2020;**12**:501

[29] Cheung K, Hume P, Maxwell L. Delayed onset muscle soreness: Treatment strategies and performance factors. Sports Medicine. 2003;**33**(2):145-164

[30] Arent SM, Senso M, Golem D, McKeever K. The effects of theaflavin-enriched black tea extract on muscle soreness, oxidative stress, inflammation, and endocrine responses to acute anaerobic interval training: A randomized, double-blind, crossover study. Journal of the International Society of Sports Nutrition. 2010;**7**(1):11

[31] Ahmadinejad Z, Razaghi A, Noori A, Hashemi SJ, Asghari R, Ziaee V. Prevalence of fungal skin infections in Iranian wrestlers. Asian Journal of Sports Medicine. 2012;**4**(1):29-33

[32] Kordi R, Mansournia MA, Nourian RA, Wallace WA. Cauliflower ear and skin infections among wrestlers

in Tehran. Journal of Sports Science and Medicine. 2007;**6**(CSSI-2):39-44

[33] Alaranta A, Alaranta H, Helenius I. Use of prescription drugs in athletes. Sports Medicine. 2008;**38**:449-463

[34] Clavel T, Desmarchelier C, Haller D, Gérard P, Rohn S, Lepage P, et al. Intestinal microbiota in metabolic diseases: From bacterial community structure and functions to species of pathophysiological relevance. Gut Microbes. 2014;**5**:544-551

[35] Zhang C, Zhang M, Wang S, Han R, Cao Y, Hua W, et al. Interactions between gut microbiota, host genetics and diet relevant to development of metabolic syndromes in mice. ISME. 2010;**4**(2):232-241

[36] David LA, Maurice CF, Carmody RN, Gootenberg DB, Button JE, Wolfe BE, et al. Diet rapidly and reproducibly alters the human gut microbiome. Nature. 2014;**505**:559-563

[37] Aguirre M, Eck A, Koenen ME, Savelkoul PH, Budding AE, Venema K. Diet drives quick changes in the metabolic activity and composition of human gut microbiota in a validated in vitro gut model. Research in Microbiology. 2016;**167**(2):114-125

[38] Nicholson JK, Holmes E, Kinross J, Burcelin R, Gibson G, Jia W, et al. Host-gut microbiota metabolic interactions. Science. 2012;**336**(6086):1262-1267

[39] Anghel M. The link between gut microbiota and athletic performance. EC Nutrition. 2019;**14**(4):322-328

[40] Salarkia N, Ghadamli L, Zaeri F, Sabaghian Rad L. Effects of probiotic yogurt on performance, respiratory and digestive system of young adult female endurance swimmers: A randomized controlled trial. Medical Journal of The Islamic Republic of Iran. 2013;**27**(3):141-146

[41] Lima dos Santos A, Cardoso Jorge AO, Soléo Ferreira dos Santos S, Silva CRGE, Pereira Leão MV. Influence of probiotics on *Candida* presence and IgA anti-*Candida* in the oral cavity. Brazilian Journal of Microbiology. 2009;**40**(4):960-964

[42] Fayock K, Voltz M, Sandella B, Close J, Lunser M, Okon J. Antibiotic precautions in athletes. Sports Health. 2014;**6**(4):321-325

[43] Bhattacharyya N, Kepnes LJ. Associations between fatigue and medication use in chronic rhinosinusitis. Ear, Nose, & Throat Journal. 2006;**85**(8):510, 512, 514-515

[44] Wosinska L, Cotter PD, O'Sullivan O, Guinane C. The potential impact of probiotics on the gut microbiome of athletes. Nutrients. 2019;**11**:2270

[45] Huang WC, Hsu YJ, Li H, Kan NW, Chen YM, Lin JS, et al. Effect of *Lactobacillus plantarum* TWK10 on improving endurance performance in humans. Chinese Journal of Physiology. 2018;**61**:163-170

[46] Townsend J, Bender D, Vantrease W, Sapp P, Toy A, Woods C, et al. Effects of probiotic (*Bacillus subtilis* DE111) supplementation on immune function, hormonal status, and physical performance in division I baseball players. Sports. 2018;**6**:70

[47] Pyne DB, West NP, Cox AJ, Cripps AW. Probiotics supplementation for athletes—Clinical and physiological effects. European Journal of Sport Science. 2015;**15**:63-72

[48] Huang WC, Lee MC, Lee CC, Ng KS, Hsu YJ, Tsai TY, et al. Effect of *Lactobacillus plantarum* TWK10 on exercise physiological adaptation, performance, and body composition in healthy humans. Nutrients. 2019;**11**:2836

[49] Nay K, Jollet M, Goustard B, Baati N, Vernus B, Pontones M, et al. Gut bacteria are critical for optimal muscle function: A potential link with glucose homeostasis. American Journal of Physiology. Endocrinology and Metabolism. 2019;**317**:E158-E171

[50] Okamoto T, Morino K, Ugi S, Nakagawa F, Lemecha M, Ida S, et al. Microbiome potentiates endurance exercise through intestinal acetate production. American Journal of Physiology. Endocrinology and Metabolism. 2019;**316**:E956-E966

[51] Ni Lochlainn M, Bowyer R, Steves C. Dietary protein and muscle in aging people: The potential role of the gut microbiome. Nutrients. 2018;**10**:929

[52] Hughes RL. A review of the role of the gut microbiome in personalized sports nutrition. Frontiers in Nutrition. 2020

[53] United Nations, Department of Economic and Social Affairs, Population Division. World Population Ageing 2017—Highlights (ST/ESA/SER. A/397); 2017

[54] Flevari A, Theodorakopoulou M, Velegraki A, Armaganidis A, Dimopoulos G. Treatment of invasive candidiasis in the elderly: A review. Clinical Interventions in Aging. 2013;**8**:1199-1208

[55] Kauffman CA. Fungal infections in older adults. Clinical Infectious Diseases. 2001;**33**(4):550-555

[56] Bongomin F, Gago S, Oladele RO, Denning DW. Global and multi-national prevalence of fungal diseases-estimate precision. Journal of Fungi. 2017;**3**(4):pii: E57

[57] Falagas ME, Apostolou KE, Pappas VD. Attributable mortality of candidemia: A systematic review of matched cohort and case-control studies. European Journal of Clinical Microbiology. 2006;**25**(7):419-425

[58] Silva S, Negri M, Henriques M, Oliveira R, Williams DW, Azeredo J. *Candida glabrata*, *Candida parapsilosis* and *Candida tropicalis*: Biology, epidemiology, pathogenicity and antifungal resistance. FEMS Microbiology Reviews. 2012;**36**(2):288-305

[59] Barchiesi F, Orsetti E, Mazzanti S, Trave F, Salvi A, Nitti C, et al. Candidemia in the elderly: What does it change? PLoS One. 2017;**12**(5):e0176576

[60] Zaremba ML, Daniluk T, Rozkiewicz D, Cylwik-Rokicka D, Kierklo A, Tokajuk G, et al. Incidence rate of *Candida* species in the oral cavity of middle-aged and elderly subjects. Advances in Medical Sciences. 2006;**51**(1):233-236

[61] Hof H, Mikus G. *Candida* infections in the elderly. Zeitschrift für Gerontologie und Geriatrie. 2013;**46**(1):64-70

[62] Rusu A, Randriambelonoro M, Perrin C, Valk C, Álvarez B, Schwarze AK. Aspects influencing food intake and approaches towards personalising nutrition in the elderly. Journal of Population Ageing. 2020

[63] Trif M, Muresan L, Bethke M. Personalised nutritional powder for elderly developed in optifel european project. Bulletin UASVM Food Science and Technology. 2016;**73**(2):149-150

[64] Guo X, Li J, Tang R, Zhang G, Zeng H, Wood RJ, et al. High fat diet alters gut microbiota and the expression of Paneth cell-antimicrobial peptides preceding changes of circulating inflammatory cytokines. Mediators of Inflammation. 2017;**2017**:9474896

[65] Fulop T, Larbi A, Dupuis G, Le Page A, Frost EH, Cohen AA, et al.

Immunosenescence and Inflamm-aging as two sides of the same coin: Friends or foes? Frontiers in Immunology. 2018;**8**:1960

[66] Khanna S. Microbiota replacement therapies: Innovation in gastrointestinal care: Microbiota replacement: An innovation. Clinical Pharmacology and Therapeutics. 2018;**103**(1):102-111

[67] Aw D, Silva AB, Palmer DB. Is the thymocyte development functional in the aged? Aging (Albany NY). 2009;**1**(2):146-153

[68] Le Couteur DG, McLachlan AJ, de Cabo R. Aging, drugs, and drug metabolism. The Journals of Gerontology. Series A, Biological Sciences and Medical Sciences. 2012;**67**(2):137-139

[69] Deray G. Amphotericin B nephrotoxicity. The Journal of Antimicrobial Chemotherapy. 2002;**49**(1):37-41

[70] Pfaller MA, Diekema DJ. Epidemiology of invasive candidiasis: A persistent public health problem. Clinical Microbiology Reviews. 2007;**20**(1):133-163

[71] Clark TA, Slavinski SA, Morgan J, Lott T, Arthington-Skaggs BA, Brandt ME, et al. Epidemiologic and molecular characterization of an outbreak of *Candida parapsilosis* bloodstream infections in a community hospital. Journal of Clinical Microbiology. 2004;**42**(10):4468-4472

[72] Gajdács M, Dóczi I, Ábrók M, Lázár A, Burián K. Epidemiology of candiduria and *Candida* urinary tract infections in inpatients and outpatients: Results from a 10-year retrospective survey. Central European Journalof Urology. 2019;**72**(2):209-214

[73] Osawa K, Shigemura K, Yoshida H, et al. *Candida* urinary tract infection and *Candida* species susceptibilities to antifungal agents. The Journal of Antibiotics. 2013;**66**:651-654

[74] Hills RD Jr, Pontefract BA, Mishcon HR, Black CA, Sutton SC, Theberge CR. Gut microbiome: Profound implications for diet and disease. Nutrients. 2019;**11**:1613

[75] Lewis JD, Chen EZ, Baldassano RN, Otley AR, Griffiths AM, Lee D, et al. Inflammation, antibiotics, and diet as environmental stressors of the gut microbiome in pediatric Crohn's disease. Cell Host & Microbe. 2015;**18**:489-500

[76] Llewellyn SR, Britton GJ, Contijoch EJ, Vennaro OH, Mortha A, Colombel JF, et al. Interactions between diet and the intestinal microbiota alter intestinal permeability and colitis severity in mice. Gastroenterology. 2018;**154**:1037-1046

[77] Chiba M, Abe T, Tsuda H, Sugawara T, Tsuda S, Tozawa H, et al. Lifestyle-related disease in Crohn's disease: Relapse prevention by a semi-vegetarian diet. World Journal of Gastroenterology. 2010;**16**:2484-2495

[78] Lewis JD, Abreu MT. Diet as a trigger or therapy for inflammatory bowel diseases. Gastroenterology. 2017;**152**:398-414

[79] Hoffmann C, Dollive S, Grunberg S, Chen J, Li H, Wu GD, et al. Archaea and fungi of the human gut microbiome: Correlations with diet and bacterial residents. PLoS One. 2013;**8**:e66019

[80] Claesson MJ, Jeffery IB, Conde S, Power SEO, Connor EM, Cusack S, et al. Gut microbiota composition correlates with diet and health in the elderly. Nature. 2012;**488**:178-184

[81] Cottier F, Tan AS, Xu X, Wang Y, Pavelka N. MIG1 regulates resistance of *Candida albicans* against the fungistatic effect of weak organic acids. Eukaryotic Cell. 2015;**14**:1054-1061

[82] Allonsius CN, Van Den Broek MFL, De Boeck I, Kiekens S, Oerlemans EFM, Kiekens F, et al. Interplay between lactobacillus rhamnosus GG and *Candida* and the involvement of exopolysaccharides. Microbial Biotechnology. 2017;**10**:1753-1763

[83] Cozma-Petruț A, Loghin F, Miere D, Dumitraşcu DL. Diet in irritable bowel syndrome: What to recommend, not what to forbid to patients! World Journal of Gastroenterology. 2017;**23**(21):3771-3783

[84] El-Salhy M. Diet in the pathophysiology and management of irritable bowel syndrome. Cleveland Clinic Journal of Medicine. 2016;**83**:663-664

[85] Auchtung TA, Fofanova TY, Stewart CJ, et al. Investigating colonization of the healthy adult gastrointestinal tract by fungi. mSphere. 2018;**3**(2):e00092-e00018

[86] Naglik JR, Gaffen SL, Hube Bf: Discovery and function in *Candida* albicans infections. Current Opinion in Microbiology. 2019;**52**:100-109

[87] Bethke M, Muresan L, Trif M. OPTIFEL personalized calculator. Bulletin UASVM Food Science and Technology. 2016;**73**(2):151-152

[88] Dietrich T, Carmen Villaran D, Velasco M, Echeverría PJ, Pop B, Rusu A. Crop and plant biomass as valuable material for BBB. Alternatives for valorization of green wastes (book chapter). In: Biotransformation of Agricultural Waste and by-Products: The Food, Feed, Fibre, Fuel (4F) Economy. Elsevier; 2016. DOI: 10.1016/B978-0-12-803622-8.00001-X

[89] Basso PJ, Câmara NOS, Sales-Campos H. Microbial-based therapies in the treatment of inflammatory bowel disease—An overview of human studies. Frontiers in Pharmacology. 2019;**9**:1571

[90] Wilson D. A tale of two yeasts: *Saccharomyces cerevisiae* as a therapeutic against candidiasis. Virulence. 2017;**8**(1):15-17

[91] Zangl I, Pap IJ, Aspöck C, Schüller C. The role of lactobacillus species in the control of *Candida* via biotrophic interactions. Microbial Cell. 2019;7(1):1-14

[92] Ishikawa KH, Mayer MP, Miyazima TY, Matsubara VH, Silva EG, Paula CR, et al. A multispecies probiotic reduces oral *Candida* colonization in denture wearers. Journal of Prosthodontics. 2015;**24**(3):194-199

[93] Kohler GA, Assefa S, Reid G. Probiotic interference of *Lactobacillus rhamnosus* GR-1 and *Lactobacillus reuteri* RC-14 with the opportunistic fungal pathogen *Candida albicans*. Infectious Diseases in Obstetrics and Gynecology. 2012;**2012**:636474

[94] Aarti C, Khusro A, Varghese R, Arasu MV, Agastian P, Al-Dhabi NA, et al. *In vitro* investigation on probiotic, anti-*Candida*, and antibiofilm properties of *Lactobacillus pentosus* strain LAP1. Archives of Oral Biology. 2018;**89**:99-106

[95] Peneluppi Silva M, Rossoni RD, Campos Junqueira J, Cardoso Jorge AO. In: Rao V, Rao LG, editors. Probiotics for Prevention and Treatment of Candidiasis and Other Infectious Diseases: Lactobacillus spp. and Other Potential Bacterial Species, Probiotics and Prebiotics in Human Nutrition and Health. Rijeka: IntechOpen; 2016. DOI: 10.5772/64093

[96] Buggio L, Somigliana E, Borghi A, Vercellini P. Probiotics and vaginal microecology: fact or fancy? BMC Women's Health. 2019;**19**:25

[97] Martínez Y, Más D. Role of Herbs and Medicinal Spices as Modulators of Gut Microbiota [Online First]. Rijeka:

IntechOpen; 2020. DOI: 10.5772/intechopen.91208

[98] Santos VR, Pereira EMR. Antifungal activity of Brazilian medicinal plants against *Candida* species, *Candida Albicans*, *Doblin Sandai*. Rijeka: IntechOpen; 2018. DOI: 10.5772/intechopen.80076

[99] Sam QH, Chang MW, Chai LY. The fungal Mycobiome and its interaction with gut bacteria in the host. International Journal of Molecular Sciences. 2017;**18**(2):330

[100] Rusu AV, Penedo BA, Schwarze AK, Trif M. Smart Technologies for Personalized Nutrition and Consumer Engagement (Stance 4health Eu H2020-Funded Project). Bulletin UASVM Food Science and Technology. 2020;**77**(1):97-100